Real-Life Healthy You

Obtaining and Maintaining Health

Shannon Simmons

Doctor of Health Sciences

A Real-Life Healthy You

You can write to the author at ssimmons@corban.edu.

To my dedicated husband, Tyrone, who has encouraged and put up with all of my nutrition and fitness antics; who meets me at the end of finish lines and cheers me on to pursue my dreams. To my beautiful children, Olivia, Preston, and Taysom, who give me motivation to be a better person. I love you all.

Your past is not an excuse for what you are, it's an explanation.

Now let's move on and make tomorrow better!

Thanks to my dear friend and amazing photographer Donny Zavala for helping make this book user-friendly with photos!

Contents

INTRODUCTION

The world of health and fitness is an ever-changing landscape. A decade-full of elliptical machine, cardio-crazed vegetarians is often followed by a decade of weight lifting carnivores—and everyone claims their strategy is the best at getting lean and staying fit. It can be terribly frustrating and difficult for the average American to determine which way is up. Do I juice? Detox? Lift heavy weights or lift light ones?

This bouncing back and forth between the goods and evils of health is leaving us more obese than ever.

Millions of people suffer the devastating effects of obesity and disease, including diabetes, hypertension, and heart disease. But when the average American family is stretched to their limit with sports practices, homework, and commuting to work, there is very little time left to focus on health, let alone research what we are all supposed to do to get healthy. Over the past 100 years, our society has morphed from hard working, heavy labor farm work to cubicle desk jobs and hours sitting in the car. We are forced to make a conscious effort to get our daily physical activity because our daily lives do not require it from us. We have gotten busy checking Facebook and posting photos of our pets on Instagram and, whether we like to admit it or not, technology has sucked time away from us that we do not have. We claim to be lacking time for exercise and meal preparation yet the average American picks up their mobile once every 6 minutes.

Gone are the days of kid's paper-routes and bicycling to school and we've arrived at the days where kids spend more time in front of a computer or television screen than they do getting physical activity. Adults are not any better, spending much of their time also sitting behind a screen and not preparing meals, but heading through a fast food line.

Whether you're a gym rat or a couch potato, there are always ways to make your life a bit healthier on the inside and the outside. This book will offer ways to get a great workout at home or in the gym. We'll look at gadgets that help us in our busy lives and ways to make eating nutritiously a bit easier. No one needs a deprivation diet or the perfect workout. We will discuss cardiovascular training for the lifespan and how to tone up for that high school reunion. Prevention of injuries is also an important area of emphasis because when people get hurt, they often have a difficult time getting back into a routine. We will also discuss creating a budget for your health; investing now in your health could save you thousands later.

I hope to answer questions in a way that is applicable; that gives you tools to take into your life immediately. We need to be myth busters and people who choose to make small changes that last a lifetime.

Many questions will be answered and topics will be explored on the hunt for what are long-lasting changes we can make in our lives and the lives of our families.

The journey toward a healthy lifestyle is one that has been near and dear to my heart. As an only child of a terminally ill parent who passed when I was eighteen, I have since felt very passionate about doing what I can in my power to obtain and maintain wellness. Many people cannot prevent disease and illness, but all of us should take advantage of the health we do have and try to maximize it.

My passion for healthy living began in childhood, growing up in athletics and being a busy participant in extracurricular activities. My childhood activity level set the stage for a life of healthy living but that was just the beginning.

Wanting to help others obtain a healthy lifestyle, I chose to study pre-physical therapy in my undergraduate studies and obtained my Bachelors of Science in Exercise Science from Willamette University in Salem, Oregon. I immediately began working as a personal trainer at a Courthouse Athletic Clubs, enjoying the personal relationships I created and helping foster healthy lifestyles in my clients. However, I began to notice a constant issue: the yo-yo of gym going and dieting. This led so many people down the path of weight gain and weight loss that they just couldn't maintain. Many clients would struggle to diet long enough to see results or would become frustrated with the slow-to-show results in their fitness regimen. People would join the gym in January only to drop their membership or just quit coming by March. They would start a diet like the Atkins diet and quickly quit because they couldn't handle the deprivation much longer.

I personally began trying different means of being the healthiest I could be. I tried bodybuilding for a couple of years. I found that this wasn't the healthy lifestyle I wanted my children to see modeled in me because I was becoming obsessive about my eating and exercise routine to the point that relationships suffered.

I have tried supplements and countless bars and shake mixes. But in the end I have found that natural, whole foods and a moderate exercise routine over a long period of time is what has led to the healthiest lifestyle that is good for me and my family.

I later obtained a Master of Science in Exercise Science and then a Doctor of Health Science degree. I now teach as a professor in the Exercise Science department at Corban University, in Salem, Oregon. I have also written for Salems's Statesman Journal Newspaper for eleven years and have been lucky enough to write for a few magazines along the way too. I continue to learn new ways and strategies to exercise from close friends and trainers, Aaron Hague, Matthew Turnquist, and Sam Mclean. I rely on experts like Susan Gallagher to give me tips for marathon training, and I've even learned great tricks from my college students. I presented nationally on research I have conducted on childhood obesity and physical self-perception as it relates to physical activity.

There is not just a single factor to blame for the health and obesity crisis in America-but there are many things we can do as individuals to improve our quality of life. If we all do a few small things, our bodies, families, nation, and world could be a healthier place.

CHAPTER 1

CARDIOVASCULAR EXERCISE

MONITORING YOUR HEART RATE

Cardiovascular exercise requires your heart rate to remain elevated. Yet heart rate intensity is one of the hardest factors to control and monitor during exercise. There are many different ways you can measure intensity including percent of maximum heart rate, rate of perceived exertion, percent of oxygen consumption, percent of heart rate reserve, and the talk test. These are just the main ones that are used in medical and fitness facilities today!

So how do you know which method to use and at what number or percentage is correct? There is a lot of recent research being done to determine what is acceptable and valid.

One of the most common used formulas and methods is the percent of maximum heart rate. You can calculate your maximum heart rate with this formula: maximum heart rate = 220-age. This formula was created in 1938 and is still used today. This formula assumes that the average persons' maximum heart rate decreases an average of 5 to 7 percent per decade. Yet recent research shows that this overestimates the change and that maximum heart rate actually declines at a rate of 3 to 5 percent per decade. Therefore you will overestimate the change of heart rate and when you determine your percent of maximum heart rate it might very well be too low for your fitness level. The typical trainer and exerciser would compute maximum heart rate = 220-age and then take that number and multiply by the range of 60 to 85 percent to find the appropriate training zone. Again, this method might give you a heart rate that is too low for you. It would not hurt you to use this formula but it is definitely not accurate. It can be extremely off with a large deviation between individuals.

The next measurement can be rate of perceived exertion (RPE). It is a number scale that matches up to your feelings of exertion. The original Borg Scale is a scale from 6 to 20 with the appropriate level being between 12 and 16; indicating moderate to high intensity. The newer version is a scale from 1 to 10 with 1 being complete rest and 10 being impossible effort. The appropriate range would be between 6 and 8 or 9, depending on your exercise goals. This scale works well but only if you are honest with yourself as to how hard you are working. Often times we believe we are working harder than we actually are, especially if we are new to exercise and are naturally uncomfortable pushing ourselves.

A more medical way to measure heart rate is a percent of maximal oxygen consumption or VO2 max. One would have to go through a graded exercise test to determine your maximal oxygen consumption and then find the percentage range of 50-85 percent of that.

Another common method is called the Karnoven formula, which uses your heart reserve to determine your training heart rate. The great thing about this formula is it allows you to take into account your resting heart rate, which varies greatly from person to person. The Karnoven formula is a step above the other formulas since each person's fitness level varies and can be somewhat exhibited in their resting heart rate.

Let's assume you want to find your training heart rate at 60 percent your heart rate reserve (HRR). Use your measured maximum heart rate (with an exercise test) or using the 220-age formula and also measure your resting heart rate first thing in the morning before you get up and get moving. Then plug the numbers into this formula: = 0.60 (Maximum heart rate – Resting Heart rate) + Resting Heart Rate. You could then use the same formula and substitute 0.85 for the 0.60 and you would have a range of heart rates to exercise within.

The latest research by Gellish, Golsin, and Olsen in 2007 (published in the Medicine and Science in Sports and Exercise journal) provides a new formula. They found the overestimate of maximum heart rate change with age and accounted for it in this new formula: MHR = 207 – 0.7 x age. You can then use your percentages of 60 to 85 percent of that.

To increase your stamina and ability to exercise harder, you have to exercise at the higher end of your heart rate zone. To measure your heart rate accurately you can try a heart rate monitor during exercise. Machine heart rate monitors are often wrong and inaccurate so your own personal heart rate monitors can be the best way to go. With a personal heart rate monistor, you can also measure your heart rate during daily activities.

If you are on beta-blockers, ACE inhibitors, or some calcium channel blockers for heart or blood pressure problems you might find that you cannot increase your heart rate very high even at extreme efforts. This means your medication is doing what it is supposed to do and preventing your heart from racing too fast.

If you are still confused, then just make sure you are working hard while you're exercising. You should break a sweat and have a hard time talking in lengthy sentences with someone next to you.

After exercising, cool down for at least five to ten minutes to allow your heart rate to slow and let your blood redistribute throughout your body and not pool in your lower extremities.

QUITTING SMOKING

It's no secret that smoking is dangerous for your health and that smoking is one of the hardest habits to break. However, it's a habit worth giving up for your body's sake, especially when it comes to your cardiovascular health.

When you smoke, your body's metabolic system is elevated, including increased heart rate and increased blood pressure. This can sometimes cause an elevated caloric expenditure—which will then decrease after quitting—so exercise is a great substitute. The increase in metabolic rate is from the nicotine which travels in your blood stream, causing an increase in the release of adrenaline and increasing your heart rate. This increase in heart rate can put you at a higher risk of a stroke.

Many chemicals in cigarettes circulate in your body and continue to affect the physiology of it for at least six to eight hours after you finish the cigarette. When you smoke, many physiological effects are taking place.

Smoking causes a high amount of inflammation in your airways and bronchioles so this often limits your ability to exercise intensely. Once you stop smoking, inflammation should decrease and your ability to breathe in oxygen will be improved. Exercise is a great way to increase your metabolic rate, increasing caloric burn, and improving health. If you are worried about gaining weight after you quit smoking, exercise can help prevent that.

After quitting smoking, ease into your cardiovascular exercise. Remember, that if you have not been exercising and have been smoking, your body and circulatory system are not accustomed to this time of stress (exercise). Start with just a short duration, such as twenty minutes at a low intensity (such as a walking pace) to get your body used to it. After a week or two of this type of pace, you can slowly increase your walking pace and try to extend your time to thirty or more minutes. If you feel short of breath, slow down or take a short break, then get back to it. Aim to get at least three days of exercise a week. Once you feel like you are accomplishing this goal, increase your frequency by adding another one or two days. Also, try a variety of exercises so that you find one you will enjoy. The warmth and humidity of a swimming pool might be good for those who have breathing problems in dry air. And if you need to, you could start on a bicycle if circulation in your legs is limited.

Be kind to yourself. Quitting smoking is a huge success and if you have been fairly sedentary, it will take time to increase your fitness levels. The good news is that quitting smoking will immediately cause improvements in your pulmonary and cardiovascular systems—so take it one day at a time. Think positively about all that you have accomplished and how each day is a step to a healthier you.

RUNNING

Beginning Running

Starting an exercise program is never a fun thing to do and does not always feel good. In fact, it only takes a few weeks of detraining to start to feel the effects when you hit the road again. This can be true of any exercise and when you are just starting out you will feel sluggish, tired, and fatigued much sooner.

The things that you can expect when you are starting are shortness of breath within the first ten to fifteen minutes with increasing exertion, increased heart rate, and increased breath frequency. These physiological responses are normal when you are pushing your body past what it is accustomed to. If you are getting burning in your chest, have a dry cough, or fatigue with dizziness you could be showing signs of something more severe.

The first disease that you could be showing signs of is asthma. The National Heart, Lung, and Blood Institute (NHLBI) reports that signs of asthma are coughing that is often unproductive (little phlegm), wheezing (a squeaky sound when you breathe), chest tightness, and shortness of breath (often a feeling of not being able to push air out of your lungs). There are many different triggers to asthma and different people respond differently to different stimulants. Common stimulants include allergens such as dust, pollen, grasses, and flowers. If you are used to being indoors and not exercising, the coupled effect of exercising outdoors with all of the allergens and being deconditioned could lead to a higher risk of an asthma attack. If you are prone to allergies, then consider exercising indoors to reduce triggers and seeing your physician for an inhaler prescription.

Exercise induced asthma brings about the same signs and symptoms as listed above but is often triggered by exercise. Exercise of any form can often lead someone into an asthma attack and is exacerbated by a dry, cool environment. You could also see your physician for an inhaler and consider exercising when it is more humid and warm.

Lastly, chest pains and tightness could be a sign of more serious problems such as cardiovascular disease. If you have high cholesterol and high blood pressure, get cleared by your physician prior to starting an exercise plan. In fact, if you have a cardiologist, it is recommended to undergo a stress test to determine any underlying cardiovascular disease prior to beginning a vigorous exercise program. Signs and symptoms of cardiovascular disease are also shortness of breath, chest pain, and fatigue. See your physician if you have any of these major signs and if you have been diagnosed with high blood pressure.

If you are clear of any diseases, you should avoid an overly aggressive program to start. Make sure you gradually increase your intensity by about 5 percent each week. Stay hydrated and well-nourished before your workout so you have plenty of energy to get you through the workout. It is always safe to exercise with another person, carry your cell phone, and let someone know where you are headed if you are out jogging.

Barefoot vs. Shoe Running

There are many barefoot running advocates out there now! When Australian 2:42 marathoner Michael Warburton wrote an article called, "Barefoot Running" in 2001, the rage began. His argument was based on the fact that the extra weight of the shoes could slow you down. In addition, many Olympic gold medalists in the marathon have come from countries where running barefoot was how they trained. Barefoot running can go back to 1960 when an Ethiopian runner won gold in the marathon, running barefoot in 2:15:17! One could go on and on showing incredible times of runners who have ran and trained barefoot.

What could be the physiological advantage of running barefoot? Well, we all have hundreds of muscles in our lower limbs and feet that are there for appropriate adjustments and performance in most any physical situation. In addition, we all have what are called proprioceptive mechanisms that provide feedback to our spinal cord and brain, which then send messages to other muscles and ligaments on how to adjust. An argument lies that when you put an artificial shoe on a foot that is already designed to endure most activities, you are manipulating the system; that you are somehow interfering with the proprioceptive abilities you have.

In other words, when you put on socks and shoes, your body's ability to measure and gauge the environment, forces, and various stresses is diminished. So if our ancestors ran around hunting and gathering in bare feet or very thin moccasins, does this change the need for shoes now? Yes! The problem when we assume that we have a great physiological system in our feet (which we do to an extent) is that we do not perform everyday tasks barefoot anymore. We go through our lives, starting at a very young age, wearing shoes and depending on them to provide support and protection. So if we went out and started running without shoes, we could pay severe consequences. In fact, many people as they get older have problems with their feet including plantar fasciitis from wearing heels or other badly formed shoes.

So we cannot compare ourselves to our great, great, great-grandfather who lived most of his life without shoes on and then would go run barefoot. The same thing is true for people in other countries who live most of their lives without shoes on and then can train running barefoot. If you aren't sure, think about the last time you walked on the beach barefoot for a long walk. Did your feet hurt afterward? Were your calves sore? Most likely you felt some serious repercussions from walking barefoot. Your feet are not used to this type of serious workout.

So for the majority of us, it would have been best if our feet were strengthened and trained to use their proprioceptors from a very early age (and that we not wear high heels, ladies). But the truth is our feet are most likely not built for a high intensity run sans shoes. You might enjoy being barefoot and have no problems trying some simple exercises with no shoes. However, if you have ever had foot, ankle, or low back problems, quickly engaging in barefoot workouts might not be a good idea. You might be better off buying a high-performance tennis shoe that provides the support and stability your feet need.

Some people like to run somewhere between supported footwear and barefoot; they can turn to a shoe like the Nike Free. This type of shoe was designed to provide some benefits of running barefoot but with some protection. A big warning here would be that if you have severely flat feet or dropped arches, you might need supportive shoes and possibly inserts more than another person.

Be your own judge but be very careful when you first start performing activities barefoot. It is not worth hurting yourself in the long run. Some track coaches have started training their athletes during agility drills and balance activities barefoot to engage proprioceptors without aggravating the joints that could be pounding during long distance events without shoes. There are many levels of barefoot running and activities that one could try without going to all barefoot activities.

Distance Running and Sudden Death Risk

In the past fifteen years, there have been more reports in the news of sudden death in long distance runners. With these increasing media reports, people are concerned that training for and participating in running events could put them at risk for cardiac arrest and sudden death. So is this risk a real concern?

The New England Journal of Medicine published an extensive report in 2012 on this very topic. Here are some background statistics that help us better understand the changing landscape of distance running. In 2012, 2 million people competed in a marathon, compared to just 1 million in 2010. Therefore, there has been an exponential increase in those participating in longer distance running events. An organization called The Race Associated Cardiac Arrest Event Registry (RACER) was created and designed to look at the increasing reports of cardiac arrest and cardiac dysfunction following an event like a marathon. They looked at studied cases of cardiac arrest that occurred during the running or at the finish-line recovery area within one hour after the completion of a marathon (26.2 mi) or half-marathon (13.1 mi) over the course of ten years. Of the cases of cardiac arrest in their study, causes varied from hypertrophic cardiomyopathy to anatomical cardiac abnormalities. They identified fifty-nine cardiac arrests, forty in marathons and nineteen in half-marathons, among 10.9 million registered race participants. The average age of runners with cardiac arrest was forty-two, plus or minus thirteen years. The overall incidence of cardiac arrest was one per 184,000 participants (0.54 per 100,000).

The American Heart Association reports that among all Americans, each year 424,000 people experience cardiac arrest and nine out of those ten people die. Therefore, there is much controversy as to whether the people who suffer cardiac arrest after a strenuous event such as a marathon would have incurred a cardiac arrest with activity regardless of the race and had pre-existing factors that put them at heightened risk.

The New England Journal of Medicine concludes that risk translates into 0.2 cardiac arrests and 0.14 sudden deaths per 100,000 runner-hours at risk, using average running times of four and two hours for the marathon and half-marathon, respectively. So cardiac arrest event rates among marathon and half-marathon runners are relatively low, as compared with other athletic populations, including collegiate athletes (1 death per 43,770 participants per year), triathlon participants (1 death per 52,630 participants), and previously healthy middle-aged joggers (1 death per 7,620 participants). These data suggest that the risk associated with long-distance running events is equivalent to or lower than the risk associated with other vigorous physical activity.

Many scientists believe that regular exercise can reduce your risk of cardiac arrest due to lower risk factors that lead to cardiac arrest such as plaque build-up, heart weakness, and blood flow abnormalities. Exercise is a positive way to lower risk of a cardiac event, but caution must be taken to identify your possible risk.

Pre-participation exercise testing with your physician may be useful for identifying some persons at high risk. Also, it is wise to obtain a full physical examination prior to undergoing strenuous exercise such as marathon training. If you have any diagnosed heart problems, you should consult your physician prior to participation. If you have any risk factors such as high blood pressure, high cholesterol, are currently sedentary, smoke, are obese, or have a first degree relative who has died of a cardiac event under the age of fifty-five, you should seek physician screening prior to participation.

RACING

Relay Racing

Running relay races can be the most fun runners have during the racing season! Fun, competition, and lots of runner-minded people make for a fun atmosphere and can be much different than running a single race. Besides the difference in training frequency and intensities that lead up to a relay, preparation reaches into many areas. When preparing for a relay, the captain is usually responsible for the logistics of having enough team members, having vans if they are necessary, the registration, and any other major items such as lodging or volunteers needed. So what else is there to think about before a relay? A lot!

Most relays have the same basic principles: a team of twelve runners (more or less) is assembled where each person runs a few legs that span an extended period of time. This is much different than preparing for a marathon where the runner can eat a pre-race meal and take off, finishing a few hours later and can grab another meal that can be fully digested. During a relay you are running more than once within a limited number of hours. Most likely, a typical relay runner will run three legs in about thirty-six hours.

The hardest part about a relay race is the off-and-on again nature of a relay. Running at maximum intensity and then sitting in a cramped van for hours will do damage to those legs and make you feel tight and sluggish. To limit muscle cramping and stiffness, it is best to stay well-hydrated, well-nourished, and stretch those legs whenever you get a chance. Drink water often and have an electrolyte solution to drink after each leg you run. Make sure to have nutritious foods such as bananas, whole wheat bread with turkey, peanut butter sandwiches, and other easy to grab, easy to digest foods. Be cautious not to fill up on too many energy bars as this can cause gastrointestinal distress and make you feel worse come run time. Eating something your system is not used to will most likely cause backlash in your stomach and could make your run miserable.

If you have a chance to jump out of the van every time there is a runner exchange, stretch those legs. Any type of movement can lessen muscle cramping and stiffness so get out and stretch when possible. Susan Gallagher, co-owner of Gallagher's Fitness Resources in Salem, Oregon, suggests bringing a "go-with-the-flow" attitude. There will be bumps in the road (literally) and not everything will go as planned so be ready to adjust and enjoy the race.

So what will you need to be fully prepared? The lists below are a mixture of what various relay sites suggest as well as great suggestions from Susan Gallagher. Many relay race coordinators have great resources for offering ideas for what to pack as well.

Susan Gallagher suggests that your personal items should fit nicely into a small bag. If you carry too much with you, then that means less room for bodies to stretch and recover between legs. So be courteous of everyone on your team by taking up a small amount of space with personal items.

The group as a whole should have the following items at their disposal:

- Headlamp
- Flashlights w/extra batteries
- Stop watch and pencils
- Relay handbook
- First Aid kit
- Antibacterial soap (for all those port-a-potties)
- Extra garbage bags
- Items to fix a flat tire
- Vaseline
- Bug spray
- Painkillers such as Tylenol and ibuprofen
- Icy Hot
- Instant ice packs
- Scissors
- Ace bandages
- Tarp
- Paper towels
- Noise maker or device in case of emergency and needing help
- Reflective tape
- Reflective vests

The individual runner should consider packing:

- A set of running wear for each leg, PLUS an extra set (t-shirt, shorts, pants, socks)
- Extra pair of running shoes (it might be wet out and you will need a spare pair)
- Extra socks for between legs to keep your feet warm and dry
- Flip-flops to air your feet out
- Warm up pants for between legs
- Electrolyte replacement
- Safety pins for bib numbers
- Sunglasses
- Deodorant
- Toothbrush and toothpaste
- Soap and shampoo
- Two to three towels and washcloths
- Lip balm
- Personal medications
- A small cooler full of lots and lots of EASILY digestible food (this is not the time to try new foods–take what you like and what will easily digest)
- Spending money
- Cell phone and car charger
- Camera
- Music
- Sleeping bag or blanket and pillow
- Hand wipes

Precautions and Preparations for Long Distance Events

- Follow a training program that allows for very gradual increases in intensity and mileage. This will reduce your risk for a sudden event.

- Get a full physical examination, including a stress test if you have any high risk factors (high blood pressure, high cholesterol, smoker, live a sedentary lifestyle, or have a first degree relative with history of a heart attack).

- Listen to your body. Enjoy participating in the race without pushing your body to an uncomfortable intensity.

- Wear a heart rate monitor to monitor your variations in heart rate during training and racing.

Marathon Training

Many people think that finishing a marathon is out of their reach but you would be surprised how easy it can be to accomplish if you have a plan and the baby steps to get you there. More than 250,000 Americans run marathons each year. There are more than 500 marathons to choose from each year and many of the runners are recreational runners, not the highly competitive types. So this could be your year to accomplish the great bucket-list item that is finishing a marathon!

The very first thing you should do is consult your physician and make sure they give you the green light to train for and compete in a marathon. Most of the hard work will be done in the weeks leading up to the marathon so also make sure to have the support of your spouse, partner, friends, and/or family. It can be very helpful to have a large team of supporters when you need encouragement for your long training runs and at the event itself!

Most marathon training guides suggest that a new runner have the ability to run a 10K before you sign up for a marathon. However, you can always sign up for a marathon way out in the future and also a 10K in about three months as a stepping stone to the marathon. Many marathon training programs are at least sixteen weeks in length. Some very experienced marathoners can gear up in a bit shorter time and some programs can last longer if you are serious beginner. But the minimum amount of time when training for a marathon is sixteen weeks.

A typical marathon training programs consists of tempo runs, interval runs, hill repeats, and a long, slow duration run. It can be very helpful to sign up with a marathon program that gives you very specific training days. Daily email reminders about what your next day or two of training is supposed to be helps keep you accountable and allows you to not think too hard about the details.

16-Week Marathon Training Schedule

Week	Mon	Tue	Wed	Thu	Fri	Sat	Sun	Total
1	3	Rest	4	3	Rest	5	Rest	15
2	3	Rest	4	3	Rest	6	Rest	16
3	3	Rest	4	3	Rest	7	Rest	17
4	3	Rest	5	3	Rest	8	Rest	19
5	3	Rest	5	3	Rest	10	Rest	21
6	4	Rest	5	4	Rest	11	Rest	24
7	4	Rest	6	4	Rest	12	Rest	26
8	4	Rest	6	4	Rest	14	Rest	28
9	4	Rest	7	4	Rest	16	Rest	31
10	5	Rest	8	5	Rest	18	Rest	36
11	5	Rest	8	5	Rest	12	Rest	30
12	5	Rest	8	5	Rest	20	Rest	38
13	5	Rest	8	5	Rest	10	Rest	28
14	5	Rest	8	5	Rest	22	Rest	29
15	3	Rest	5	3	Rest	8	Rest	19
16	3	Rest	3	Walk 2	Rest	26.2	Rest	34.2

A typical training program, like the one offered on marathonguide.com, page 28, can be a good basic start to getting you ready in 16 weeks:

- You will notice that in the training plan you do not actually run the full 26.2 miles until race day. That is okay. The adrenaline and excitement will get you through it!

- Try incorporate running various routes on your middle of the week runs so that your legs are used to a variety of terrains and elevation changes.

Different Types of Training Runs

Tempo Run: After warming up with a slower paced jog for ten minutes, you want to amp up your speed just to slightly below race pace and sustain that intensity for at least twenty minutes. Then slow yourself for the last ten to fifteen minutes of your training time. You could perform this twice a week. Tempo runs are great at increasing your stamina and ability to run faster for an extended period of time.

Hill repeats: If your race might have some hills in it, you must incorporate this. Hill repeats are also good for anyone trying to increase their work capacity. Warm up for five to ten minutes. Find a hill that is 100 to 200 meters long and one that will push you but not force you to change your form. Push hard up the hill at your 5K pace and then walk down. Repeat this two to eight times, depending on your fitness ability. You want to keep your gaze ahead of you, not at your feet, to insure you are maintaining good form.

Interval workouts: Warm up for ten minutes at an easy jog and then speed up to about 80 percent of your race pace. Run at this intensity for four minutes and then increase your pace to almost race pace for three minutes. Then slow back down for four minutes. Continue repeating this interval style for the majority of your assigned miles, slowing down one to two miles prior to completion to finish.

Taking Time Off After Racing

The length of time you take to taper before a race and the time you take to recover after a race is largely dependent on the distance you ran. For a shorter race, such as a 5K, you might not need as much recovery time, especially if you did not run to your maximum intensity. If you are running a longer distance such as a half or full marathon, you will need a fairly decent taper before and after your race.

Before a distance such as an 8K, you could begin to taper the intensity and distance you run a week or ten days prior to your race. You will not lose your strength and endurance in a week's time. So if you are going to race on a

Sunday, then you should probably have your last long run the Saturday before. If you are running a marathon, or even a half-marathon if you are a beginner, then you could do a gradual taper two weeks prior to the race. Two weeks prior to the race, do your last long run. Then do three days a week of lower intensity and fewer miles each day. You want to keep your muscles moving and loose but not to the point of exhaustion. So get your hill and fartlek days of training in before you begin the taper. Fartleks are a method of training that includes continuous running with bursts of speed work throughout.

After a race, again it largely depends on the distance and your experience level. If you are a seasoned runner and run a short race you might need less time to recover before hitting the road again. However, if you just ran your first marathon you might want to take a week or two off from running before training hard again. It can take some time for new running legs to recover from the distance and intensity of a marathon. The best way to gauge how much time off you need is by how you feel. If you are extremely sore, then you might want to take enough time to be able to maintain good form.

Your rest and recovery time should be active. Active recovery involves moving your body at a lower intensity that does not jar your body to the degree that the race did. Try swimming for your cardiovascular workouts or do lower intensity cycling. Another focus could be on something such as yoga or guided stretching to lengthen your muscles and recover.

Another important factor of recovery is sleep and nutrition. After a race, you can feel like you now deserve to eat junk for a week. A celebratory meal is great fun but don't let your nutrition fall for a week or more after the race. You will not feel like hitting the road again if you have only filled yourself with junk. Plus, your muscles need healthy carbohydrates and lean protein to recover and prep for another bout of training. Sleep is also crucial. Your body repairs during sleep, so your nightly shut-eye should equal at least eight hours on the nights leading up to and after a race for adequate muscle recovery.

If you enjoyed your race, then sign up for another one. Give yourself enough time in between the two to recover and feel good for the second race. It is good to have a goal race to reach for and something to train for.

BICYCLING

Most people love being outdoors when the weather brightens up after a cold winter. Bicycling is a wonderful cardiovascular activity to enjoy in the great outdoors. The benefits of cycling are the non-impact, non-weight bearing aspects of this form of exercise. You can get great exercise with very little joint irritation and get fresh air at the same time. But what if you only hop on your bike between June and August? You tend to be sore and often unprepared.

Cycling will feel better if you are already in good physical condition. It is a good idea to achieve balance, core strength, flexibility, and cardiovascular health prior to hitting the road. So before you jump on your bike for a long ride, I suggest you approach this activity like you would any other cardiovascular exercise. You need to work your mileage and intensity up slowly. Try cycling some indoors to strengthen your leg and lower back muscles. Try to cycle at least two days a week to build up strength and endurance. Like other forms of cardiovascular exercise, you should warm up and cool down after a workout and also stretch!

I even suggest trying a spinning class at a local health club. Your body can be well conditioned with a spinning class and this can transfer over into outdoor cycling. Plus, a spinning class offers great instruction on form and provides motivation to push your body beyond what you might attempt alone. Riding a bike on the road will require much more core strength and balance than a stationary bike does, however you could start training in the gym by riding a stationary bike in order to increase your cardiovascular stamina.

Other indoor things you can do to prepare for outdoor cycling are core exercises. Try to perform three different abdominal and lower back exercises on three non-consecutive days each week. A strong core will prevent low back pain and increase your stamina. Core exercises will also improve your balance. Try the following for core strength and flexibility:

- Standing balancing on one foot for thirty seconds. Progress by closing your eyes and raising arms up and down to the sky ten times.

- Planks – hold for thirty seconds. Add alternating hip extensions to advance exercise. By keeping leg straight and lifting up higher than hips while squeezing the buttocks.

- Chest stretch in a doorway – hold for thirty seconds. Find a doorway and put shoulders and elbows at 90 degrees, resting forearms on the doorjamb. Gently lean into the doorway as to stretch your pectoral muscles.

- Hip bridging. Lie on your back with knees bent. Keeping your hips level, raise your hips towards the sky, hold for ten seconds and repeat. Advance by lifting one foot off the ground.

Bicycling is a very popular activity for recreation, physical activity, and even transportation. If you're new to cycling, the League of American Bicyclists offers many resources. To begin, it is good to check your ABC's. A stands for air; are your tires inflated properly? B stands for brakes; make sure your bicycles' brakes are tested. And C stands for cranks, chains, and cassette; make sure to get these all checked out at your local bike shop before you hit the road. If you're shopping for a bicycle, be sure to visit a local bicycle store for assistance in picking out a good bike for your use, your level, and body size.

Many local bicycle shops offer group rides for all ability levels so contact one in your area for the next opportunity to ride with a group. Riding with a group can encourage you, offer insight to the sport, and allow you to learn from those who have participated longer. As well, riding with a group can be a safe way to get out on the road for a beginner.

Before heading outdoors on your bike, you should run through a checklist of items. You should first have a bicycle that suits your body and the type of cycling you will do. Will you be racing, riding on the road, or biking on trails? Utility bicycles are used for errands and commuting. Touring bicycles are often used for long journeys. They are more comfortable and have a wider gear range. Cruiser bicycles have ballooned frames and look like what was popular in the 1950s. They are very comfortable but are not built for speed. If you are looking for speed and ride on the road, you could look into a racing bike. They are lightweight and have very high gear options. Go to a reputable bicycle shop to get the best advice and help in purchasing a bike that suits your needs.

Consider purchasing a small tire pump that you can carry with you in case of emergencies as well as a small bicycle bag that can carry identification, a cell phone, and any medication if you need it. If you are planning on cycling far, you might want to have clips installed on your pedals and buy special cycling shoes. This will help you go faster for longer! Finally, you definitely need a water bottle to keep you well hydrated.

Make sure you know the path you are riding. Try not to go out alone if you are in a secluded area and tell someone where you are going and when to expect you back. I also suggest not cycling in the dark. If you have to ride in the dark to commute to or from work, you should have a very well lit bicycle and wear many reflectors on your clothes.

The League of American Bicyclists offers a fun "Ten Commandments of Bicycling":

I. Wear a helmet for every ride and use lights at night

II. Conduct an ABC Quick Check before every ride

III. Obey traffic laws: ride on the right, slowest traffic farthest to right

IV. Ride predictably and be visible at all times

V. At intersections, ride in the right-most lane that goes in your direction

VI. Scan for traffic and signal lane changes and turns

VII. Be prepared for mechanical emergencies with tools and know-how

VIII. Control your bike by practicing bike handling skills

IX. Drink before you are thirsty and eat before you are hungry

X. Have fun

GARDENING AND YARD WORK

If you do a lot of gardening or yard work, you know how it can make your body feel stiff and sore. In fact, gardening and yard work may feel terribly excruciating, especially for those of us whose bodies are not used to that type of work year round. But is it actually enough of a workout to substitute for your normal exercise routine?

In an hour, your body burns around 250 calories planting, 350 calories hoeing, and up to 500 calories if you are doing some serious digging. Of course this number varies depending on your body weight and how hard you are working. If you are mowing your yard with a push mower, you could burn upwards of 400-500 calories depending on how large your yard is! This calorie burn is as much as you might burn in a typical aerobics class. You are definitely burning enough calories doing yard work to justify skipping that morning walk. However, the type of activity you are getting is much different than a typical gym workout.

When performing yard work, you are risking low back pain and injury. This is one of the biggest reasons people should continue their normal—and probably more intense—core exercise. If your core musculature is weak going into a Saturday of gardening, then you are setting yourself up for a low back injury. With all of the leaning over, slouching, and digging done in a typical day of gardening, you are putting your back in a very vulnerable position. This slumped over position is already flexing your spine in a way that is putting discs in a compromised position. If you have a weak low back and abdominal region you could hurt yourself with one wrong move.

Therefore, continue to perform a weight training routine at least two days a week and train your core (abdominals, low back, buttocks, and hips) at least three non-consecutive days a week. One great exercise for your core is the quadruped: kneeling on your hands and knees, back flat, lift one hand and the opposite leg simultaneously and hold for five seconds while keeping your spine straight and abs in. Repeat going back and forth from side to side ten times.

To further work your core, perform abdominal crunches on a stability ball. Instead of curling your shoulders toward your knees, lift your chest up toward the sky: do two sets of twelve repetitions.

For your low back you can also perform a Pilates move called swimming. Lying on your stomach, pull your abdominals in and then lift both arms and legs. Quickly raise higher one hand and the opposite leg simultaneously without holding. Instead of pausing, lift opposite sides back and forth for a total of twelve times. Continue to breathe throughout all repetitions.

A simple way to strengthen your core is to maintain proper spinal alignment during your daily activities. Make sure your pelvis doesn't rock forward or backward as you walk around, work on your computer, or do dishes. Contract your abdominals and keep the following landmarks aligned: ears, shoulders, hips, and ankles.

All of these exercises will prepare you for even the most grueling yard work while minimizing the chance of injury. While gardening, be sure you kneel down when you can instead of stooping over and rounding your back. Get yourself a gardening stool so you can sit while weeding and move often so you are not reaching too far away.

Take a break every fifteen minutes to stretch your low back and hamstrings. This will lessen the pressure you feel on your back. While taking a break, get a big drink of water to stay hydrated.

You should also take the time to stretch after your gardening day is over. It is critical to take as little as five minutes to stretch your low back in order to release muscle tension. Lie flat on the floor and bring one knee up to your chest and hold for thirty seconds. Repeat on the other side. Then sit up with legs straight and lean forward while keeping your back flat. Hold the hamstring stretch for thirty seconds while taking deep breaths.

Enjoy the activity of gardening and being outdoors but do not ignore your overall conditioning as it can help prevent injury and reduce soreness afterward!

WATER EXERCISE

Exercising in the water isn't simply limited to swimming laps. In fact, water aerobics and various forms of water exercise are great ways to gain a lot of physical strength, endurance, flexibility, and stamina. As well, water aerobics can vary in intensities and provide a valuable exercise experience for all ages and levels.

The Center for Disease Control (CDC) states many benefits of water exercise. Just two and a half hours per week of aerobic physical activity—such as swimming—can decrease the risk of chronic illnesses (ie. diabetes, heart disease, high blood pressure). The CDC states that water exercise reduces the symptoms of rheumatoid and osteoarthritis such as stiffness, swelling, and loss of range of motion. They also state that it can help decrease anxiety and depression in those suffering from fibromyalgia and improve quality of life and decrease disability for the elderly.

Exercise in water has also been reported to be more fun than that on land, and this can be especially true with all of the variety of water classes available. Water provides a great place to increase your range of motion since the buoyancy of the water can help assist your limbs in moving further—and usually with less pain. Exercise in water can elevate your heart rate like any land exercise and is a great way to cross train if you perform other types of exercises that are more jarring to the body.

Properties of Water in our Favor

Buoyancy: Buoyancy is an object's ability to float—in this case, your ability to float. Exercise in the water minimizes the forces and pressure on joints. If you are someone who has osteo- or rheumatoid arthritis or just sore joints from too much pounding over the years, it can be beneficial to get exercise in an environment with buoyancy. The deeper you go in the water, the more body weight is taken off of your joints. For example, if you are at waist height in water, you will have about 30 percent of your body weight taken away. If you go in up to your collarbone, you will feel about 70 percent of your bodyweight taken away by the buoyancy of water.

Viscosity = Resistance: Viscosity is the extent to which a fluid resists a tendency to flow. Water's viscosity causes there to be a resistance against motion, which can increase the intensity at which we move in water. When exercising in water, you can increase the resistance by speeding up your body's movement in the water. You can also increase resistance if you are in a water class and hold an implement of some kind that would increase the water surface area you are moving. This could also be true if you wore webbed gloves. Resistance helps exercise in water feel more intense and increases the use of muscular force!

Pressure: Water exerts a pressure and the weight of water increases the pressure as you go lower. Water pressure can help improve circulation by pushing against the body and muscles. This pressure can also increase return blood flow to the heart and lungs if you are upright.

Turbulent flow: Turbulent flow is a fluid motion in which velocity, pressure, and other flow quantities fluctuate irregularly in time and space. When you hold a paddle board against the water while kicking with your feet, you see the water bubbling up and causing resistance in front of and behind the board. This will help you in the water to create increased resistance and can either help or hinder you when you are exercising or swimming laps in a pool. Your body cutting through the water from underneath to above the water demonstrates this.

There are many different forms of water exercise. You can find therapeutic aquatic classes at therapy clinics. If you are looking for a well-balanced class, try a gym class. For rhythmic classes, try water aerobics and even Aqua Zumba. With such a variety, you can be challenged in the water no matter what fitness level you are at.

Aquatic therapy is one of the best and safest forms of exercise for those who have major joint problems. If you have knee or low back pain when you exercise then the buoyancy of the water can help lessen your body weight for exercise. The water allows for a comfortable environment for you to move in, allowing you to get aerobic and resistance exercise in without the jarring and irritation on your joints.

There are many forms of aquatic therapy and you can easily vary the intensity levels to fit your situation. One of the best methods for getting the best out of your pool time is to take a water aerobics class. Classes provide instruction and motivation to exercise safely and effectively while in the water.

Most health clubs and gyms have a water aerobics class. I suggest that you check the certification of your instructor. Your instructor should have her CPR/First aid certification and specialized training in aquatic therapy.

Physical therapists are often good teachers of water exercise and know the specific limitations and exercise needs of various injuries or physical conditions. Try contacting a local physical therapist if you want some guidance in the pool.

If you are unable to attend an exercise class, then have a plan when heading into the pool. You should look at a pool workout like any other workout; it is the same as preparing for weight training. If you head to the weight room and have never used any of the equipment, you end up standing there looking confused or even possibly hurting yourself. The same is true in the water. If you don't have a plan or have not been trained in the water, you could end up not being effective or hurting yourself.

For land exercise such as cycling, walking, and jogging, your target heart rate is usually calculated as 60 to 85 percent of your predicted maximum heart rate. However, your target heart rate is lower when you are submerged in water. In fact, you should use this formula: 220-age-13 to predict your maximum heart rate for water exercise; then calculate 50 to 85 percent of that number. The reason for this is that your heart rate is naturally slower under water due to better venous blood flow return to the heart.

Once you know your target number, you can take a quick fifteen second count every ten minutes of your exercise. Multiply that number by 4 to find your heart rate.

Just as in land exercise, you should warm up before any vigorous activity. Do some easy water walking in the shallow end before beginning to swim laps or other intense activity. If swimming laps is not your idea of fun, then you can try the following exercises. If any of them are too easy, add resistive devices such as webbed gloves, foam handbells, and kickboards.

Lower body:

- Leg lifts: move legs in and out, up and down.
- Knee to chest: holding onto pool with both arms, lift knees to chest. Progress to facing away from the edge of the pool.
- Wall walks: face edge, hold on with both hands, and walk feet up side of pool.
- Flutter kicks: face down, holding onto edge of pool, perform small kicks emphasizing ankle action with little knee motion.
- Scissor kicks: either prone or supine, make large, full range kicks, up and down, in and out.
- Lunges: lunge forward and backward
- Speed Walking: walk forward and backward
- Mini-jumps: jump in place
- Mini-hops: hop in place
- Mini jumping jacks

Upper body:

- Push/pulls with kickboard or other hand held devices. Be sure to use a good support stance to maintain balance.
- Pushups on the edge.
- Big arm circles

SNOW SPORTS

Hitting the slopes is fun and a great form of physical activity, but people can risk injury if they are not conditioned. You might fall into one of these categories: you are sedentary until you put those skis on and fly down the mountain, or you are exercising but not doing the right things to get you in ski-season shape. When preparing for ski-season and other winter activities, you should incorporate cardiovascular fitness, muscular endurance, and some very important full body movements that you might encounter while skiing, snowboarding, or snow-shoeing.

So many winter sports require very sport specific athletic movements and skills. If our bodies aren't ready for these moves, and then we perform them for hours at a time, we can end up wishing we had prepared better!

If you are taking children or other beginners to the slopes, consider private lessons. If your family is new to snow sports and your children are older, then take a group lesson together and try to make it fun for everyone.

Whether or not you take lessons, consider the basic fitness level of everyone in your group before you even head to the mountain. Everyone should be able to support themselves with their leg muscles through basic endurance and strength exercises. Make sure you can all walk at least a mile and can perform some basic squats and calisthenics such as push-ups. Skiing and snowboarding can be very physically demanding sports. The more in shape you are first, the better everyone will feel during the process.

For many people who are frequent gym-goers, they often get in a rut of performing machine based lifts and elliptical trainer type movements. All of those things are great for basic fitness and health; however, when you participate in a sport of full body activity, your body needs to be prepared to respond to a variety of movements and risky maneuvers. For example, performing a seated leg extension concentrates work on the quadriceps muscle group but does little for strengthening the entire lower body as it is utilized during movements like hiking and skiing. As well, bicep curls might help tone your arms for tank top season, but don't do much for giving you better endurance and strength for the mountain.

Here are some great ideas for full body exercises that will utilize full body strength and core endurance which will help you be better prepared for the twists and turns you will encounter outdoors. Perform these exercises a couple days each week in conjunction with an adequate cardiovascular endurance program of three to four days a week of at least thirty minutes or more.

Turkish Get Up

It has a funny name, but this exercise incorporates every muscle in your body and also requires balance and coordination, which are essential in skiing and boarding. To begin, lie on your right side with a kettle ball or dumbbell in your hands. Roll to your back and allow the weight to be entirely supported by your right hand with your right arm extended straight up to the sky with your hand directly over your shoulder. Then bend your right knee and place your left hand down on the ground and extend your left leg out to start pushing yourself up. As you push yourself up bring that left leg behind you and move to the lunge position. Keeping the right hand with weight extended above your right shoulder, stand up from the lunge position. Repeat ten times on each side.

Box Jumps Front/Back and Lateral

Stand behind an eighteen-inch or higher step. Jump up on top of the box and back down. Repeat fifteen times. Rest and jump on to box from both the left and the right sides.

Wide Walking Lunge with Twist

Holding a medicine ball at your chest, step out with your right leg into a lunge. Simultaneously extend your arms with the medicine ball straight out in front of you and twist to the right. Step together and repeat with the left foot and twisting to the left. Repeat for twelve repetitions on each side.

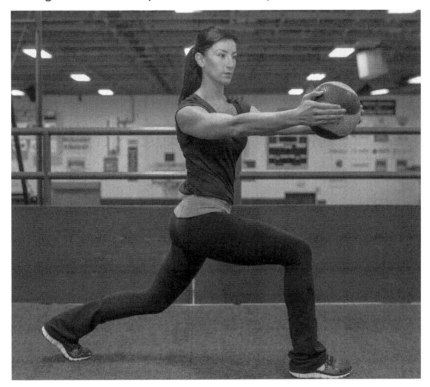

Burpees

This old-fashioned gym exercise is a great way to build up your muscle power, endurance, and cardiovascular fitness all at once. To begin, start in a push up position and drop down all the way to the floor. Then jump or step your legs into your hands. Then raise your arms up and jump as high as you can. Go to failure at the end of your workout.

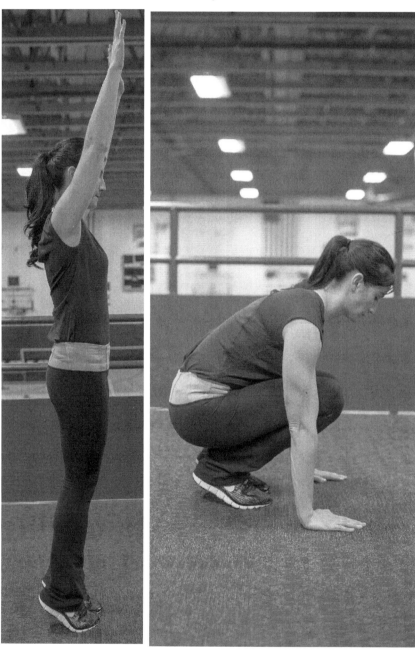

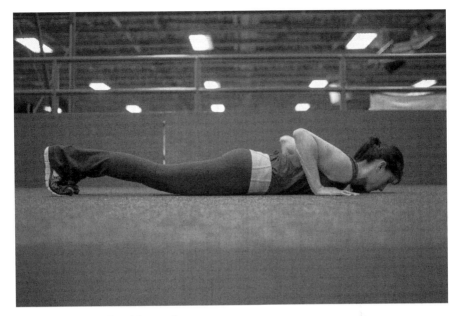

Cardiovascular Exercise

If you really want to be ready for your favorite winter activity, try to mimic the movement during your cardiovascular workouts. If you are a cross-country skier, then hop on a cross-country skiing machine like a NordicTrack®. If you like snowshoeing, then get on the Stairmaster® or rotating stair machine. For those of you hitting the slopes on skis or a board, walking or jogging on an incline could increase your lower body power.

If you can hit the gym now and get some personal training before a day or weekend of snow sports, you can build up cardiovascular and muscular stamina. If you can get a session on a vibration plate (at some local gyms and physical therapy clinics), you can improve your balance, coordination, and strength of stability ligaments. If that is too pricey for you at this time then begin some activities that will improve your strength. All of the following activities are great for involving the whole family: At least three times a week, head out before dinner for a walk around the neighborhood. You can also do some push-ups, squats, and abdominal exercises right in your living room. Effective strength training exercises include body weight or weighted squats (keeping the knees in line with your heels and not moving over your toes). You can also do walking lunges, which will help strengthen the stability muscles of your knee, decreasing the risk of injury.

Your back is an important area of core strength. Abdominal exercises are important, but without back exercises you might be creating an imbalance. Perform back strengthening exercises such as a lat-pulldown, seated row, and back extensions.

Facing a lat pull down cable machine, hold the bar wider than shoulder width. Slowly lower the bar, close to your body and right under your chin, then slowly return it to its upright position.

For the seated row, have knees slightly bent and feet firmly on the platform. Sit upright and bend elbows bringing the hands towards the stomach and pinch your shoulder blades together. Keep your shoulders down away from your ears, as to not shrug up. Focus on squeezing your shoulder blades together to work on your back muscles.

The back extension exercise can be performed on the floor. Lay face down and pull your abdominal muscles in. Extend your arms overhead and raise your upper body up off the ground. Hold for 20 seconds and repeat 3 times.

Flexibility is also a very important factor in your physical fitness and ability to recover from a hard day on the mountain. Practice some basic yoga poses and hold for thirty seconds. If you are unfamiliar with yoga then you can purchase a video for around ten dollars that can show you many poses. If even that feels too awkward, you can do basic stretches such as a forward bend, seated hamstring stretch, spinal twists, and chest stretch in a doorway. Hold each stretch for thirty seconds.
The healthier you are in general, the more fun and in less pain you will be when trying a new physically active sport.

Snowshoeing

Snowshoeing is a cardiovascular and muscular test of endurance. If you have not been accustomed to previous cardiovascular and muscular training, you will likely feel the effects of a long day out on the trails. Snowshoeing is often performed on both flat and rolling hill terrain so you should be ready to go the distance in any type of conditions. To prepare for snowshoeing season, you should aim to get miles and hours on your feet in a similar fashion. In a gym setting, aim to increase your time on the treadmill. Make sure you carry a pack on your back that is equivalent to what you will be wearing on your snowshoeing trip. As well, increase the incline on the treadmill so it emulates the conditions. For strengthening moves, add lunges since this movement mimics uphill climbing.

Snowboarding

Snowboarding is often a sport that puts a lot of stress on your lower back, thighs, and even upper body if you are a newbie and tend to fall a lot! Flexibility is also crucial due to the nature of always strapping in and out of your board so you should increase your time stretching after a workout routine. To best prepare for snowboarding, it can help you to perform exercises in a circuit fashion. Utilize your body weight for many exercises to get you ready for pushing yourself up and off the mountain.

Downhill Skiing

If it has been months since having those boots strapped to your feet, you will feel some shin soreness and pain. Try to get your legs ready for the adventure down the mountain. To prepare, aim to perform squats at least two times a week on non-consecutive days. If performing twelve repetitions with your body weight feels easy, then aim to add weight by either holding dumbbells up by your shoulders or use a bar. You can do front or back squats.

Tips for the Slopes:

- Try to warm-up beforehand. If you feel awkward doing a full warm-up and stretch before hitting the snowy slopes, you can try to ease into your activity by taking it slowly during your first twenty minutes or so. If you can find the space and time, try to stretch a little once you have warmed up.

- Don't try to be a hero. If you are new at a sport, stick to what feels comfortable to you. Injuring yourself won't impress anyone so be smart.

- If you do become sore after a day outdoors, you should move around the next day. Lying on the couch can often make your muscles stiffer and make you more miserable so try to go for a nice slow walk and stretch to get the blood moving and your muscles healing.

- Finally, make sure you are prepared out in the great outdoors, with appropriate attire to keep you warm, plenty of food and water to stay hydrated and feeling well, a way to communicate (such as a cell phone or walkie talkie) and make sure you tell someone where you are headed for the day; preferably with a buddy or partner!

REST

Do you really need to take a day off from working out—even if you feel okay without a break? A day of rest and recovery might just give you more results than exercising that day!

Here are a few things to consider. First, what type of results are you getting now? That is, if you have been working out for a while, have your results plateaued? Second, how intense are your workouts? You should really consider if you are doing the same workouts and are becoming accustomed to them. If you feel like you do not need a day of rest and recovery, then you might be exercising at an intensity that is below what would be considered overload for your body. Overload is a training principle: you have to stimulate the body into a state of overload to reap a change. That means you must overload your cardiovascular or muscular systems to see a change.

If you are at your goal weight and composition, you might be okay to continue your submaximal program to maintain your results. However, even if you are at your goal weight, you might see that over time, your body needs a change to maintain your level of fitness, weight, or composition.

Your workout should be looked at as a weeklong program, one that changes (or cycles) every month. This is called periodization—the notion that your body needs variety in mode, duration, intensity, and rest based on your goals and timing. Part of a great program, that provides physical adaptation, includes times of rest and recovery. You should be pushing yourself at a high enough intensity at least a couple, non-consecutive days a week, to warrant a day of rest. Although our bodies need exercise, they also need recovery. At minimum, most people need at least one day a week of complete rest or maybe light active rest. Light active rest could be a leisurely walk with your dog or tossing the football in the backyard with your kids.

When you rest, your body has a chance to recover. Recovery happens physically, mentally, and emotionally. Physically, your muscles need a chance to repair. The most gain in lean muscle tissue and change in body composition are accomplished during repair. Your day off could also include a light stretching if that feels good on sore muscles. Recovery also allows you to rehydrate and gain the nutrition you need to elicit change.

Mentally, without a day off, you might start to feel unmotivated and lack the ambition you once had. A day off can really help get your mind and body excited for that next workout.

Emotionally, you might need that break from exercise. If you are trying to lose weight and the pounds are coming off slowly, sometimes you can become stressed. Stress is not something you want when you are trying to lose weight because stress can often cause you to have elevated hormone levels and increase weight gain. When you have a day off, don't feel guilty that you are not exercising, but instead focus on getting great nutrients in your body for recovery (such as vegetables, fruits, and whole grains).

Another vital element in recovery is sleep. Sleep is an important factor in weight loss, lean muscle mass increase, and weight maintenance. Many people do not get enough sleep during the week and try to make up for it on the weekends. Research is conflicting as to whether you can make up for lost sleep on the weekends. Try to increase your sleep time by even fifteen to thirty minutes each evening to help muscle recovery.

CHAPTER 2

WEIGHT TRAINING

Weight training is one form of resistance exercise. Many people are fearful of lifting weights that they might get large, bulky muscles. However, it is very important that you understand that resistance training is very important for increase in lean muscle mass, increasing your metabolism, and increasing bone mineral density. The American College of Sports Medicine recommends that we do resistance exercises 2-3 non-consecutive days of the week and perform 8-10 different exercises that work all parts of the body. It is imperative that you seek professional guidance if you have not lifted weights before and if you aren't sure who to use a piece of equipment, ask a professional first. Also, resistance training can be in the form of lifting your own body weight such as push-ups, pull-ups and body weight squats. It does not require that you have a membership to a large, expensive health club, although that could help you seek the guidance you need and the variety of equipment you might want. People of all ages and abilities can perform some level of resistance exercises and see a vast improvement in strength and abilities for activities of daily living.

WEIGHT LIFTING AFTER A BREAK

For people who have done weight training in the past and now want to come back after a break, there are a few things to keep in mind. Consider the different types of muscle fibers you have: If you predominantly trained for cardiovascular fitness before taking time off, you could have had more type 1, or slow twitch muscle fibers. These types of fibers are most beneficial for long-term aerobic activity. If you lifted weights then you might have had more type 2, or fast twitch, muscle fibers; these fibers are more likely to work for short bursts of activity such as lifting weights.

With detraining, you can lose muscle (also called atrophy). What happens over a long period of detraining is the loss of your cross sectional area of muscle. The more cross sectional area, the stronger and more powerful you are. If you take time off due to a severe injury and are immobilized in a cast or splint you could lose contractile components that increase your strength.

Yet a study published in 2005 in the European Journal of Applied Physiology found that people who detrain for up to three months did not lose as much strength as expected. Thirteen sedentary men were trained for three months and found to have increased concentric (shortening of the muscle) and eccentric (lengthening of the muscle) strength after performing heavy resistance training. Then they let them detrain (completely rest) for three months and they were measured again. After the rest, the participants had similar maximal muscle strength and neuromuscular activity. So their muscles and nervous system were working similar as to before their time off. They maintained some muscle and eccentric (think the lowering phase of a bicep curl) after their time off. Their concentric strength (raising the bar during a bicep curl) was decreased.

If you've trained in the past, your nervous system likely remembers what it was like to contract those muscles; it should come back fairly easily. When returning after a long break, take it slow. Aim to do two days a week of full body weight training (about three days apart) and light cardiovascular workouts at least three days a week for about twenty minutes in duration.

When you weight train, perform just one set of ten to fifteen repetitions and make sure you move slowly and purposefully through the motion. Warm up for at least five minutes prior to lifting weights. Stretch when you are done.

When you are getting back into exercise after a break, it is best to focus on regaining muscle range of motion and endurance than absolute strength. So make sure that when you get back in the gym you practice exercises that put your body through a large range of motion.

Your diet must consist of healthy fats and natural carbohydrates to maintain muscle. Proper carbohydrates in your diet keep your body from going into a mode where it starts to waste muscle because it is not getting enough carbohydrates for energy.

TONING

One of the most common question trainers are asked is "Should I do more reps with less weight or less reps with more weight?" There are many different theories and programs out there regarding the amount of repetitions and sets you should do. It is very important that no matter how many you do, you have a method to your madness. You have to first ask what your main objectives are for working out and lifting weights. Are you looking to gain muscle mass, lose body fat, or maintain? It is also very important that you have a certified trainer show you a variety of exercises that might be effective in reaching your goals and diminishing any muscle imbalances.

Usually female clients want to look lean and tone, not necessarily bulk up. The National Strength and Conditioning Association recommends that if your goal is muscular endurance and not hypertrophy (increased muscle size), then you should do around twelve to fifteen repetitions instead of the lower range of six to ten repetitions of each exercise. The American College of Sports Medicine makes the general recommendation that most persons should perform eight to twelve repetitions of a resistance exercise for all muscle groups. The National Academy of Sports Medicine recommends increasing muscular endurance by aiming for twelve repetitions or increasing muscle size by performing eight or fewer repetitions. Most certifying organizations and research institutions would agree that there is no substantive evidence that performing extremely high repetitions does you much good when it comes to increasing muscle.

Increasing muscle will help you burn more calories throughout the day and improve your body composition, having a higher percentage of muscle and therefore, a lower percentage of fat. To increase strength, perform a weight that causes fatigue within twelve repetitions. Lifting a weight that you could perform twenty or more repetitions with will not overload the muscle enough to cause increases in strength.

When people say that they want to look more tone, they usually mean they want to decrease their body fat percentage. You have to decrease the amount of subcutaneous fat that covers up the muscle definition underneath. Much of losing excess fat is nutritive and overall caloric expenditure. So this is where higher repetitions at a fast rate come in to play. By lifting a lighter weight and performing high repetitions you might burn more calories by moving rapidly with little rest. Many new methods of higher repetition training involve performing a series of movements in quick succession without much, if any, rest. This causes your heart rate to soar and you will burn more calories than in traditional weight training. In traditional weight training—the kind you see at the gym all the time—people perform a set of twelve repetitions and then socialize in between sets. Their heart rate drops back down and they aren't burning as many calories. Instead, take a series of six or more exercises and go from one to the next with no rest. You will gain some benefit of resistance but also gain cardiovascular endurance. Your heart rate increases and if you continue working hard with very little rest, you will burn quite a few calories.

So there is not a definitive answer to the question, "How can I look more tone?" The greatest gains come from changing your routine often; keep your body guessing so that there is overload sufficient to produce physical change. If you do the same thing forever, your body will become accustomed to that and will not change. Try performing a traditional weight routine of eight to twelve repetitions for a month or two, emphasizing all of the large muscle groups to gain strength and stability. Then aim to do three weeks of interval training where you increase repetitions to fifteen and lower the weight;

perform each exercise quickly one after another without rest and see if you can tell a difference.

A very basic way to organizing your weight training program is through various phases or periods. A common term is periodization: cycling between stability, core, muscular strength, muscular endurance, and power phases. A rest phase is also often included in your half-yearly or yearly program. That being said, it is very wise to have you and your trainer plan out short term plans (perhaps a month at a time), as well as a long-term picture, that helps you map out the year or season ahead.

Lifting weights and exercising are lifelong habits and activities. If you plan to do this forever, you need to cycle in and out of various programs to be most efficient and effective. Look at your overall goal and work from there.

For most exercisers, strengthen your core first through stability and balance exercises; perform the recommended eight to twelve repetitions. If you are a beginner, you might only need one set to see a significant change.

Once you have improved your core (abs, low back, hips and glutes), start focusing on your full body. No matter which body part you are working, you can follow a basic phase pattern. Try to perform two to three weeks of each of the following formats.

For the first phase, perform supersets combining opposing muscle groups working back to back without rest. Do two exercises—such as a stability hamstring curl and the leg press—with eight to ten repetitions of three sets and then moving on to the next two superset exercises.

Then in your next phase, move to giant sets which are three or four exercises that work the same muscles from different angles. Giant sets are similar to supersets in that you do not rest in between exercises. Stick to eight to ten repetitions and three sets of each. This will increase your intensity and allow you to more easily put on muscle mass (which helps increase your metabolism and therefore lose fat). Do these types of sets for two to three weeks.

The next phase emphasizes your entire body. Once you have written either a full body program or a muscle group program you move from one exercise to the next without rest. Perform three sets but working at ten repetition maximum (using 100 percent of your maximum for ten reps). This is very intense and might not be appropriate for very beginner or injured exercisers. You are basically pushing yourself to the max each and every set and you should adjust your weight so that you can do ten full reps for each set.

Along with this format you should continue doing twenty to forty-five minutes of cardio three to five days a week. As you increase the intensity of your lifting days, you need a rest day. Your rest and recovery is just as important as your workouts!

ARM TONING

Arms are one of the easiest places to see quick results in tone because most people tend not to carry too much excess body fat in their arms. If you can start to implement some resistance training you will see very beneficial results. Of course, if you can incorporate a few days of cardiovascular training each week you will see more dramatic results because you will be burning more calories and hopefully losing any excess fat that could be hiding the muscles already on your arms!

Arm toning requires engaging all of the muscles of your arms and shoulders. The shoulder muscles can really help accentuate the shape of your arms and should not be avoided in the weight room! As well, upper body posture can really help tone your shoulders and give you the appearance of a longer and leaner upper body.

Most of the exercises given can be done at home with a few dumbbells. Aim for three, non-consecutive days of the week. Do three sets of ten repetitions with weights heavy enough that you can barely perform the last two repetitions of each set with proper form.

Alternating T's in a plank position: No weights needed

Supporting your body in a plank position with weight on your toes, legs open at a "V" and arms in a "T" with hands under your chest and arms straight. Keeping arms straight, raise one arm up and out to the side, point your thumb to the sky. This should cause you to tighten your abdominals and contract the rear portion of your shoulder. The great part about this exercise is that it works your abdominals and arms!

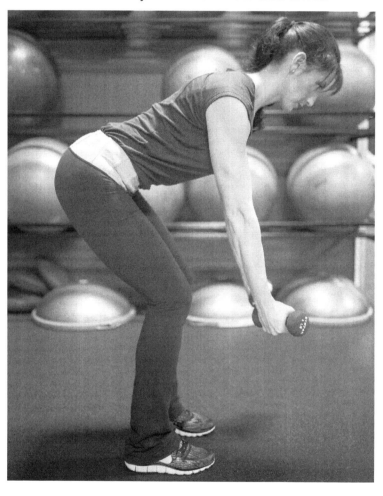

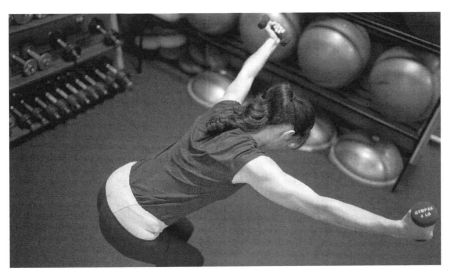

Side plank shoulder raises: Light dumbbells

In a side plank and holding body weight up with one arm and body straight, hold a light dumbbell in the top arm and keeping it straight, raise and lower it slowly up to 90 degrees at the shoulder and back down to your side.

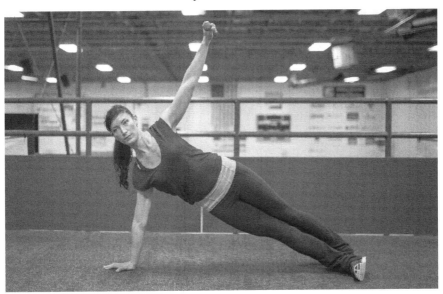

3-way bicep curls:

With arms down at your sides holding a dumbbell in each hand and palms facing forward, curl the dumbbell up and lower. Then immediately turn palms toward the sides of your legs and curl up and lower, then immediately turn palms facing down and curl the weight up. That is one repetition. Repeat the sequence of three. Make sure to keep your shoulders in good posture and elbows at your side while curling up and down.

2- way tricep extensions:

Hold a dumbbell in one hand and extend your arm straight overhead. Keeping your elbow pointed up to the sky, bend elbow and slowly lower your hand behind your head. Straighten your arm by extending hand back up. Slowly lower your hand back down with elbow still pointing up and bring hand down in front of your head. That is one repetition. Repeat for ten repetitions before switching to the other side. *See pictures on page 71.*

LEG TONING

Females naturally tend to store more body fat in their lower extremities and abdomen. This is great for bearing children, but not usually appreciated for swimsuit season. Women (and men) who desire to tone their legs can make a few changes to their workouts to get improved results.

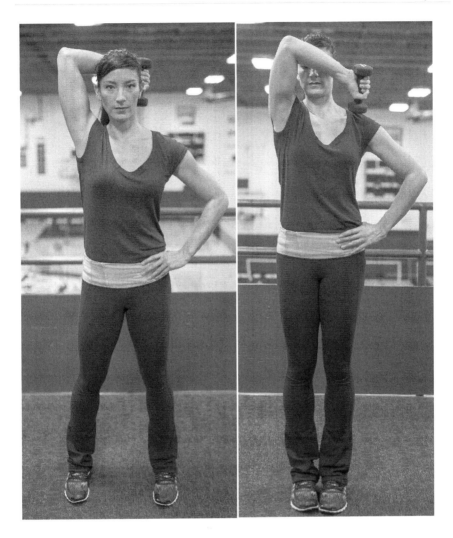

If you have been exercising in the same way for a long period of time (more than two months), change your routine to get more results. Your body will begin to adapt to the workout you are doing and will no longer change its appearance. In a way, your body says, "Oh, we do this all the time, nothing new here" and quits changing. So you need to shock the body into thinking that something new is happening and it has to keep up. To change the workout you are currently doing, ask yourself a few questions. How intense is my cardiovascular exercise? Is the resistance high enough or am I moving fast enough to burn sufficient calories? What type of resistance training am I performing? Am I doing multi-joint movements that require a lot of energy and stabilization such as squats and lunges or am I only doing isolation exercises such as leg extensions and curls? Multi-joint movements require more energy and are much more functional for everyday life.

When you do exercise that causes impact to your muscles—such as running and jumping—your muscles will pull on your bones. This strengthens your bones and your muscles slightly more efficiently than with non-impact activities. If your joints can take it, do exercises with muscle impact such as jogging or even better, plyometrics.

Plyometrics are a form of exercise where you provide maximal force with a jump or shove like movement. Most plyometrics are designed for the lower body (though you can do them for your upper body such as when performing push-ups with a clap in between). Plyometrics require a high level of energy, which translates into calories burned and an elevated heart rate, much like cardiovascular activities. They also stress the muscles in a way that stimulates more muscle development than just your basic weight lifting exercises. You can perform simple plyometrics such as jumping up onto a step and back down. You can do box jumps such as up-up-down-down or up-and-over technique. If you do not have boxes then just jumping up and down while tucking your knees to your chest will provide the same effect.

If you are new to plyometrics, perform them no more than one time per week. Plyometrics tend to really shock your muscles, bones, and tendons and require sufficient rest time. For example, if you lift weights with your lower body on Tuesday and Thursday, try adding a few plyometric exercises to your workout on Thursdays only. You should always warm up adequately to decrease your risk for injury and make sure you stretch well at the end. Plyometrics can be a great tool for shedding fat and increasing lean muscle mass to your lower body. This will not only help improve your athleticism but could tone up your legs. It is very important that you give your legs ample recovery time if you want to allow the muscle to repair. You will see great improvements in leg muscle definition.

ABDOMINAL STRENGTHENING AND TONING

Your midsection can be the hardest area to firm and tone. Women often have a much harder time seeing muscular tone in their stomachs than men do. This is due to their hereditary genes that cause more fat to be distributed there. Childbearing can also worsen the tone of the midsection. Even if you have lost the baby weight, you still have looser skin on your abdomen and that can make it difficult to see any results from hours of crunches!

Whether you're interested in looking good in your swimsuit or just wanting to have a stronger core, it's important to look at your entire workout and nutrition plan rather than putting too much faith in a few abdominal exercises. Creating and maintaining a toned midsection is a combination of cardiovascular exercise, resistance training, adequate sleep, and healthy, clean food.

Another factor that can contribute to abdominal fat deposition is stress. Some researchers believe that increased levels of stress increase your body's production of a hormone called cortisol. With small levels of stress, cortisol can help with things such as regulation of glucose metabolism, blood pressure regulation, immune function and inflammatory response. Cortisol basically helps in your fight or flight mechanism with acute stress. However, when you have elevated levels of chronic stress (e.g., from work, finances, or relational problems), cortisol can be harmful to your weight loss attempts. Negative influences of prolonged cortisol levels can be increased blood pressure, increased abdominal fat, suppressed thyroid function, decrease in muscle tissue, and lower immune system. So keep your stress in check by getting plenty of relaxation time. You can also practice deep breathing or meditation to reduce stress levels.

Nutrition is as important as exercise in decreasing total body fat. Eat three healthy meals a day and two portion-controlled snacks, all made from natural, wholesome ingredients so you can get plenty of fiber, lean protein, and healthy fruits and vegetables. Try to eat every few hours to keep that metabolism fire burning. Drink plenty of water so that you do not mistake dehydration with hunger.

Cardiovascular exercise such as walking, jogging, cycling, or swimming are very important for burning excess calories—which also helps with decreasing body fat. Aim to get thirty to sixty minutes of cardiovascular exercise on most days of the week. Cardiovascular exercise does not have to be a huge time sacrifice. Try walking for ten minutes before work, at lunch, and after work. This has been shown to be adequate in reaching your thirty minutes per day minimum.

Once you have adequate nutrition, cardiovascular exercise, and stress relief, you can focus on resistance training. Performing two non-consecutive days of full body resistance exercise will help increase total lean body mass, increase your metabolism, and decrease fat composition.

Focus on large muscle group exercises such as squats, lunges, push-ups, and pull-ups.

The benefits of a strong core go far beyond visible results. A strong core, including abdominals, lower back, hips, and buttocks, can support your spine through daily movement and activity. This reduces your risk for lower back pain and injury. A strong core can also help keep your spine in alignment and will provide a stronger body overall. Most of your strength and power comes from your core. Whether you are swinging a golf club, swimming, running, or just picking up a heavy bag of groceries, your core supports the entire movement.

Strengthening your core for functional strength can involve Pilates type movements as well as traditional core exercises. Please avoid the traditional crunch or sit-up! This type of movement is not appropriate for most people. In our daily lives, we almost never move in this type of movement with our backs supported on the floor. Crunches on the floor can actually lessen the strength of your lower back and cause back pain and weakness. Instead, opt for a less stable activity such as crunches on a physioball or BOSU® balance trainer. Your lower back should work in concert with your abdominals to be properly balanced. If you train your core functionally you will not only have stronger abs, but a stronger lower back.

The most important muscle in your core and abdominal region is the transverse abdominus (TVA). Your TVA is your own personal corset muscle that supports your spine during movement and pulls the stomach inward. To contract your TVA, practice pulling your navel in toward your spine and contract the pelvic floor muscles that would stop the flow or urination. For women this type of contraction is called a kegel exercise. Once you learn to control your TVA, you can perform exercises that improve its stability and strength.

Try pulling in your core, contracting your TVA, and holding a plank for at least thirty seconds. A plank is holding your body up off of the floor while balancing on your elbows (with forearms and hands resting on the ground) and toes.

Another exercise that is helpful is the leg drop. Lying on your back with your legs in the air, pull in your TVA and maintain a small lower back curve. Slowly drop legs toward the ground while preventing any movement at your hips or back. Only go as low as you can while maintaining no pelvic movement.

Next, try a slow bicycle crunch. Lay flat on the ground with your hips and knees bent at ninety degrees, feet off of the ground, pull your shoulders up while hands are behind your head. Open up your elbows so you are not pulling on your neck. While staying crunched up, slowly reach an elbow to the opposite knee while extending the other leg. Go back and forth until fatigued and you cannot maintain crunch. Try these exercises three days a week for improved core strength.

To strengthen the more outer walls of your abdominals, try the following exercises. Aim for twelve to fifteen repetitions and do them in a circuit fashion, one after the other and then repeating until completing two to three sets total.

- Hanging knee raises – hanging from straps around

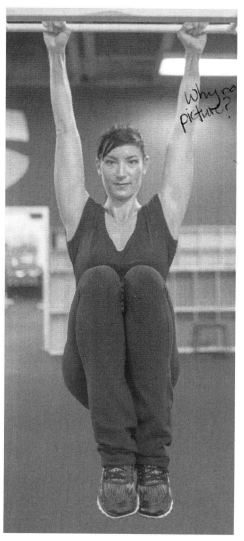

your upper arms or leaning with your elbows on a roman chair (roman chair is a piece of equipment in most weight rooms with an area of padding for your back and elbow rests), raise your knees towards your chest. Make sure you feel as if your core is doing the work, not your hip flexors. If this is too easy you can do this with straight legs.

- Weighted ball crunch – lying back on a physioball, lower back on top of the ball and legs relaxed, grab a rope attachment on a lower cable or hold a dumbbell behind your head. Raise your shoulders up toward the sky (not toward your knees) and slowly lower. Do not come all the way down where your back is hyper extending and your abs relax.

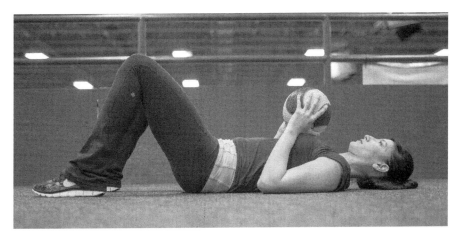

- Ball pass off – Holding a physioball or medicine ball in your hands, lie on your back. Extend your arms overhead and your legs straight out. Bring your hands and legs up over your body to form a V. Pass the ball off to between your ankles and lower back down, continuing to reach overhead with your hands. Repeat, passing the ball from hands and back down, then feet and back down to repeat repetitions. *See picture on page 80.*

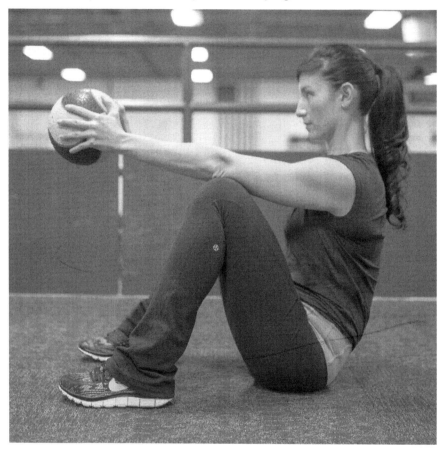

Do this abdominal circuit two to three non-consecutive days a week. After performing this circuit for a month, try to switch it up a little by substituting a different exercise or two. You should also incorporate exercises for your low back and buttocks to improve core strength.

SPEED AND AGILITY FOR EVERYONE

Speed and agility is something we often think is only for those who are ready to hit the court or field for an intense competition. However, we all need to maintain—and even increase—our speed, agility, quickness, and power. Without focusing on improving in these areas, we quickly lose our fast twitch muscles that increase our quickness and we tend to decrease our reaction time that could help in all types of life circumstances. We all need some level of power to get up and out of a chair, we need quickness to dart out of the way of someone inadvertently coming at us, and we all need speed to maintain a level of activity that keeps us young and viable. One of the biggest consequences of losing power and quickness can be an increase in a risk for falling. If you neglect your power and speed training, you risk falling and injuring yourself.

Precautions prior to speed and agility training

- If you have had a major joint injury (especially knee injuries) or surgery, get physician clearance prior to adding movements that involve directional change.

- Start slowly (use a lower step for jumping, allow yourself more time, and be patient).

- Wear appropriate footwear for shock absorption and easy directional change.

There are some basic activities that anyone can do to increase and maintain speed, agility, quickness, and power. Try to do the following exercises at least once a week.

For speed:

- At a local track, complete ten twenty-second runs at 90 percent of your maximum heart rate. After each sprint, rest for one to two minutes by walking.

- Run up stairs or an incline for ten to twenty seconds to increase your ability to speed up.

- Fartlek running: warm-up jog for five to ten minutes. Then increase your speed to a race pace for five minutes; recover by jogging at your warm-up pace. Repeat this sequence three times and cool down.

For agility:

- Play hopscotch. At a local school or playground, use painted (or draw your own) hopscotch. You can do the traditional method (2-1-2…) or try to hit each square with just your right leg and then repeat with your left.

- Find a painted parking line and do double leg hops over and back across the line for thirty seconds, as quickly as possible.

- Set up eight cones in a line and try to quickly zigzag run up and back with a shuffle step so your feet create the following pattern: Hopping back and forth (R= Right, L = Left)

For power:
- Jump with both feet up on top of a box at least eighteen inches high. If this is too high, start lower. Repeat for ten repetitions.
- Holding a five to fifteen pound dumbbell or kettlebell with your right hand, start with the weight on the ground between your legs (wider than hip-width apart), squat down with your back straight and explosively

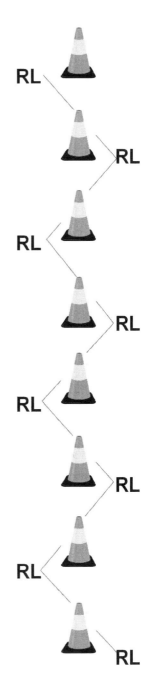

swing the dumbbell up to shoulder height. As you throw the kettlebell up your power should come from your hips as you straighten your knees and extend your hips so you are standing at the top. . Repeat six to eight times.

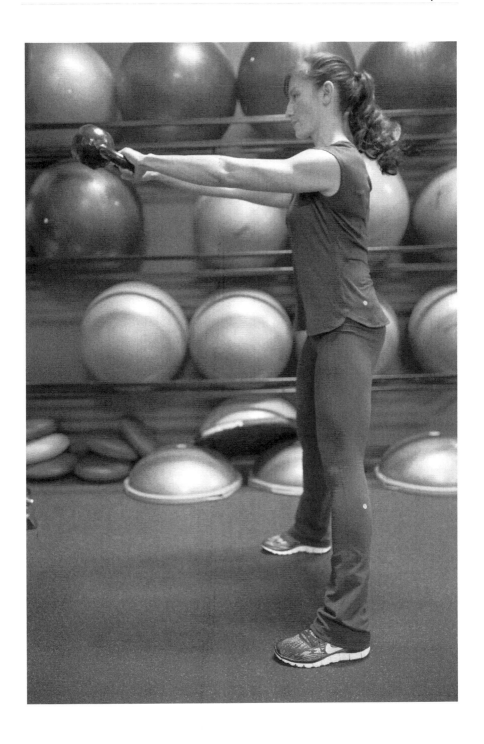

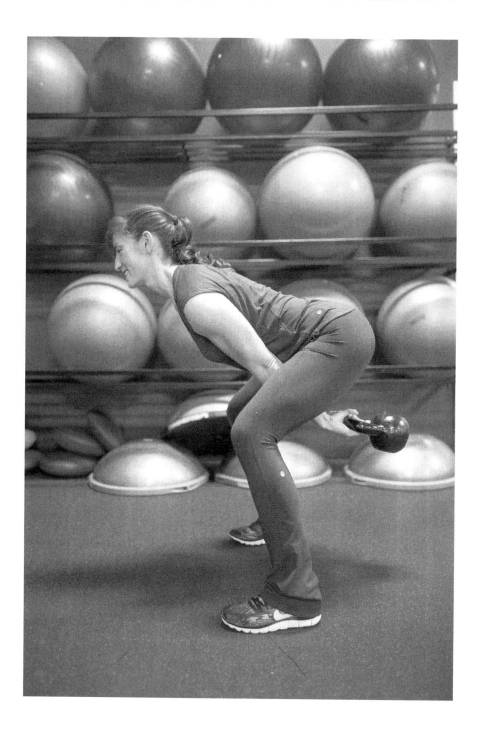

CHAPTER 3

EXERCISING AT THE GYM

Although you can easily get in all the exercise you need during the week without belonging to a gym, it can be easier to slack off when you're on your own. When people exercise in a gym, they tend to push themselves harder and stick to a plan that will reap benefits. For example, a health club membership might offer classes that you enjoy and the motivation to keep working hard. When you do cardiovascular exercise on a machine, you might be motivated to increase the minutes you have been active and therefore complete more total minutes.

HOW TO PICK A GYM

Picking the right gym for your needs can be difficult. It is often easy to pick the gym with the lowest monthly membership costs but sometimes it might benefit you to look at a few other factors.

The first thing to consider is how it suits your particular needs. Some people strictly want water aerobics classes and therefore should look at a health club that has both a pool and a water aerobics schedule that fits their personal calendars. It won't help you to sign up for a particular class if it isn't offered at a time that you can take it. Also, ask the membership associate if the class that you are interested in is something that is consistently on the schedule rather than a special class that could go away in the future. Tour the weight room to check for equipment that you particularly like using. Is the weight room terribly busy at a time that you will be using the equipment? If cardio equipment is important to you and you want to be able to watch a show or the nightly news then look to see if they have access to media.

If you are looking for hands-on personal training, then maybe a smaller training studio atmosphere will fit the bill. There are many great private facilities out there. Look for a trainer that is nationally certified and has a degree in exercise science, human movement, or a related area of expertise.

Second, look at the amenities and any extra charges. Will you want to shower at the gym before heading off to work or home? Do they charge for the use of a locker if you need one? Do you need to bring your own towel or will they charge you for towel use? Is the membership you are looking at limited to certain times of the day? Some health clubs have created windows of time that are generally lower use and offer memberships for those times of the day at a discounted rate. That could be great for you but could be harmful to consistent workouts if your workout times vary. If you are interested in a special class or area of the gym, ask if use of those areas require extra charges.

Is the gym clean? Every gym will have a little bit of dust in back corners but do they have hand disinfectant around the facility? Do the locker rooms and showers look like they have been recently mopped and cleaned? Methicillin-resistant Staphylococcus aureus (MRSA) is often found in gyms so you want to know if they clean on a regular basis.

Get details on the fine print. The great low rate might be just in the monthly dues yet they fail to let you know that there is a cancelation charge or a high initiation fee that will end up costing you a fortune. Read the details carefully before signing anything.

Another important thing to consider is the professionalism and safety of the personnel. Gyms and health clubs vary widely in the caliber and experience of the staff. The staff should be certified in CPR and first aid. A staff that is polite and trainers and instructors with professional certifications are signs that they are invested in their profession and take it seriously. If you are taking exercise advice from them then you want to be ensured that they are giving you appropriate recommendations that will better you and reduce any harm including risk to injury.

Joining a gym is a very valuable way to stay accountable and have the access to a variety of exercise equipment and classes. If staying on a consistent exercise plan at home by yourself is not working, then join a gym. Investing in your health could encourage you to stick to exercising. Plus, you will probably work harder in an environment with other people.

YOUR BEST THIRTY MINUTES IN THE GYM

We are all pressed for time and getting in a workout can feel like just one more thing on the calendar. If you have thirty minutes to work out but tend to do the same routine over and over, there is a chance you aren't getting the most out of your time. Performing the same exercises and routine month after month, year after year, is not only boring to your mind, but also boring to your body. Try to spice up your thirty minutes by incorporating new exercises and making your time as efficient as possible.

There is plenty of research out there that states that bursts of high intensity training will increase your overall caloric expenditure. This is great news for those of us who are pressed for time and could use an intense calorie burn!

For the treadmill lover:

Instead of your normal stroll on the treadmill while watching the news or your favorite TV show, try to amp it up. A thirty-minute television program is the perfect frame to plan your routine around. Every time there is a commercial, increase your intensity to a run that is fast enough so you can only speak two to three word phrases. This is usually around 85-90 percent of your maximum exertion level. You might not be able to maintain this speed during the entire commercial segment in the first few workouts, but you can work up to it!

If running is not an option for you, increase the incline/grade of the treadmill during the commercials. Whatever you do, try not to hang on to the front handrail, as that will lessen the intensity and work of walking up the hills. In the first commercial break, increase your grade by 3 percent; each consecutive commercial break go up by 2 percent more (so 3 percent, then 5 percent, then 7 percent, and so on for the show's duration).

For the weight room:

Pick six exercises that will incorporate most of the muscles of your body. For example, squats, pull-ups, push-ups or bench press, shoulder press, lunges, and planks. Perform one set of each exercise at a weight that is intense enough that you can only perform eight repetitions. After one round (set) of each exercise, head quickly to the cardio room and perform four minutes on either the bike or treadmill at an intensity that is high enough you cannot sing, but can talk in short sentences. Then head back to the weight room and complete another set of your weight training exercises. This workout will help you fit in your resistance moves while keeping your heart rate up which will help you burn more calories and fit in both cardio and weights!

Before we move into the pictures, I want to add: Be sure to catch the "For the pool" section on page 102. Thanks!

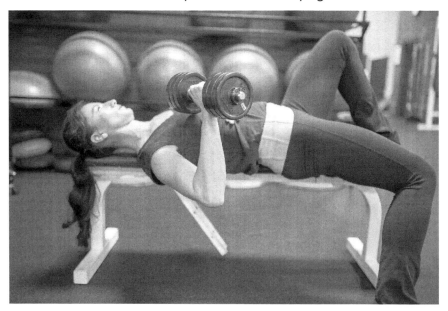

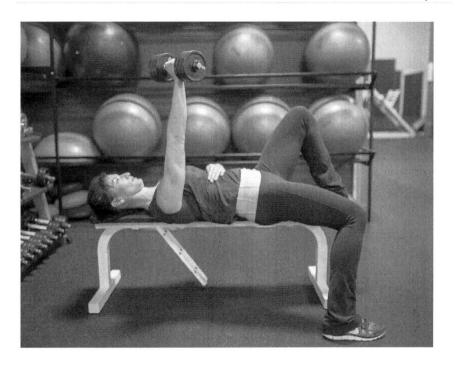

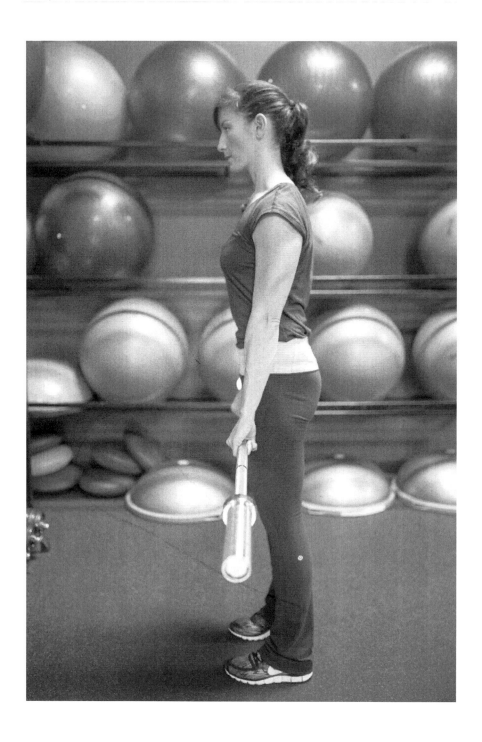

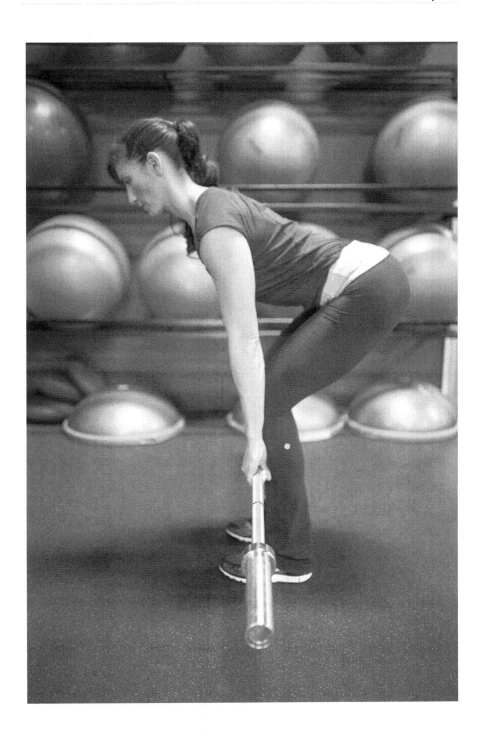

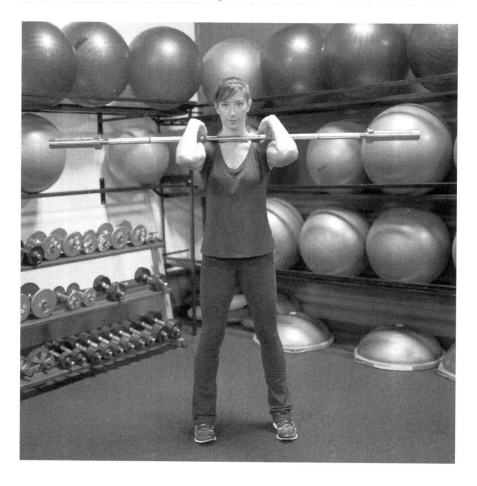

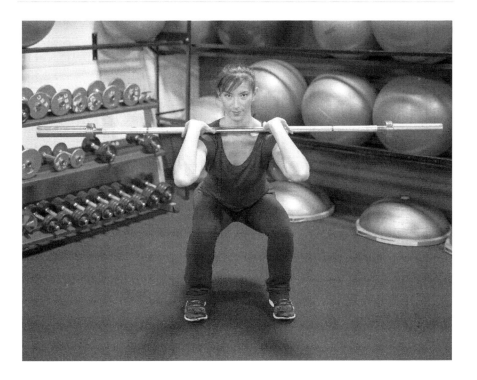

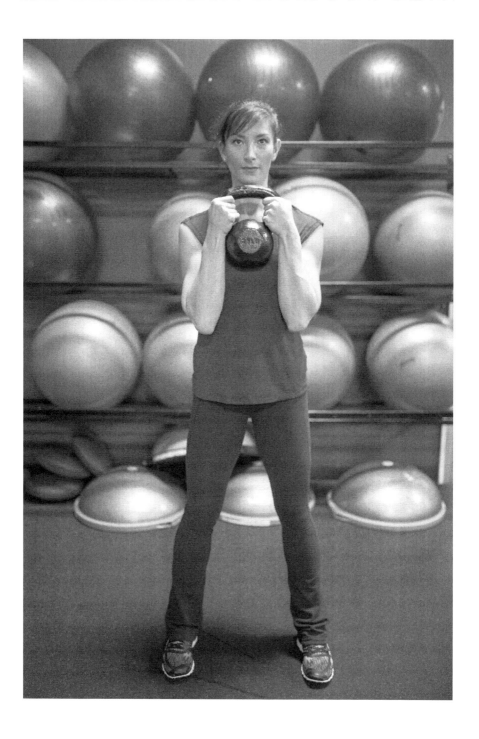

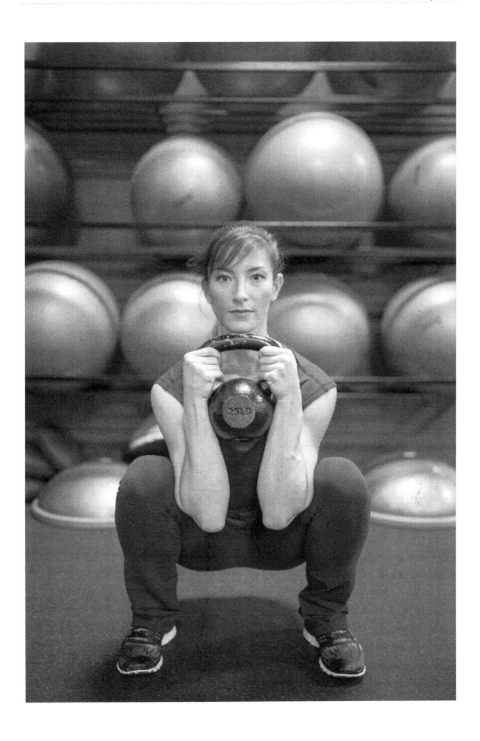

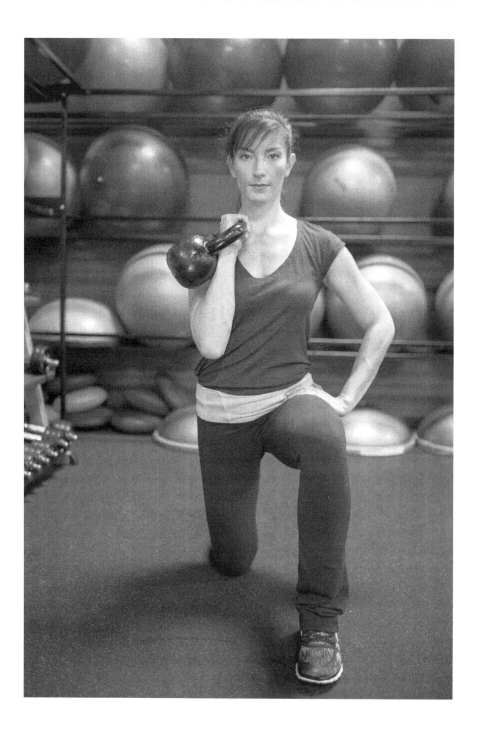

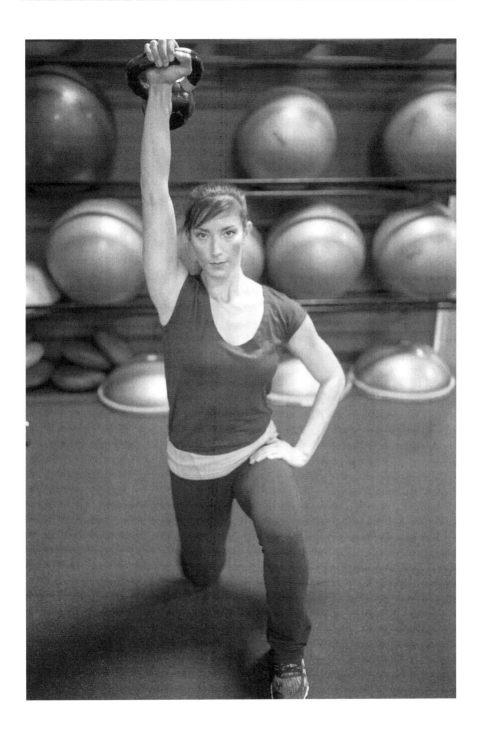

For the pool:

Break up your normal pool routine into segments. The ideal way to divide up a thirty-minute workout is to do ten minutes of warm-up, fifteen minutes of the main set, and five minutes of cool down. Depending on your swimming ability, you may cover anywhere from 1,000 to 2,500 meters, so the workout below has room for variation according to your ability (this plan covers 1,800 meters).

Warm-up:

300 meters (five minutes)

4x50 kick/swim (individual medley order: fly, back, breast, free) (five minutes)

Main Set:

400 meters (5.5 minutes)

300 meters (4.75 minutes)

200 meters (3 minutes)

100 meters (1.5 minutes)

Cool down:

300 meters (backstroke, breaststroke) (5 minutes)

CHAPTER 4

EXERCISING WITHOUT A GYM

Having a gym membership is helpful for keeping your exercise routine but of course you can exercise without a membership! The important idea behind exercise is to increase your physical activity, caloric expenditure, strength, and overall health. You can do all of those things without a gym. Just be careful that you still give your body the intensity and duration of exercise minutes it needs to maintain or possibly improve your strength and fitness.

If you are interested in exercising but an investment in personal training or a gym membership seems too steep, then there are ways you can write your own exercise program. In the internet age we are in, you can find some reputable sites that can assist you in developing an exercise program. Whether it's a book, website, or personal trainer, the most important thing is finding a source that is reputable and carries licensure or certification. Look for an exercise program that blends a realistic amount of cardiovascular, strength, and flexibility exercises.

Before planning your various exercises, think about scheduling your weekly exercise plan. If you are a beginner, then plan to do three days of exercise. A great program could be a Monday, Wednesday, Friday program that each involve some sort of cardiovascular and resistance training component. If you can be exercise for an hour, then plan on thirty minutes of resistance training and thirty minutes of cardiovascular activity. As a beginner, you want to do a simple full body routine that will get your body's metabolism up and help teach your nervous system how to perform the exercises properly.

A full body resistance training program should consist of exercises for the following body parts: core (low back, abdominals, and glutes), legs, back, chest, shoulders, and arms. If you are new to weight training, then do one set of eight to twelve reps for each body part.

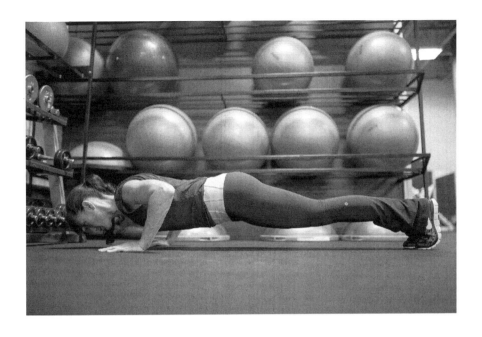

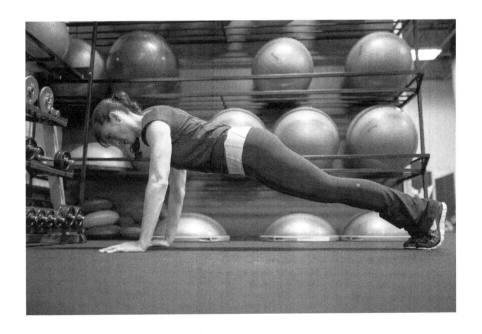

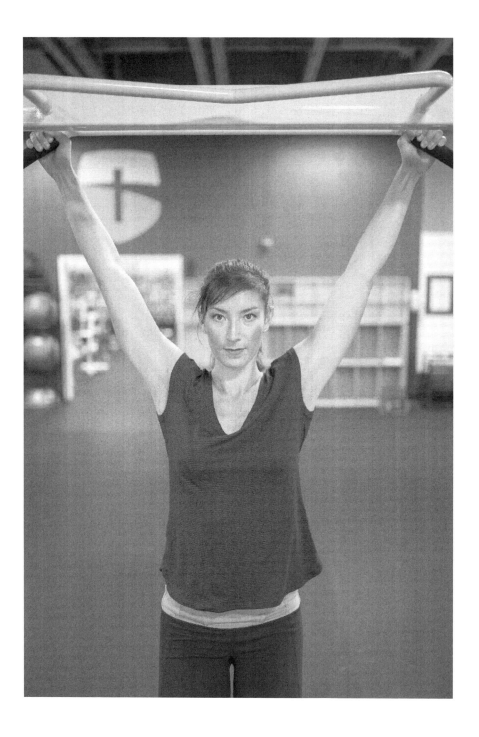

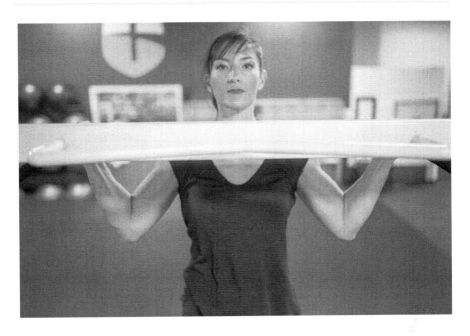

Another tactic is doing full body exercises that incorporate your entire body at once instead of splitting them up individually. So instead of doing a squat and then a shoulder press separately, you could do them together. These types of compound exercises increase your body's energy demands and can aid in balance and core strength.

Create a workout log on a sheet of paper. Write down in the left column what body part each exercise will focus on. On the right side, track your exercise days and workouts. As always, before beginning your weight training, you should warm up for at least five minutes.

SIMPLE EXERCISES ON THE GO

Think of all of the ways you *could* move and yet don't. The basic health recommendation is to reach 10,000 steps (or five miles) of walking a day to improve your overall health. If you get up and walk, that might be a good start in your mission to increase physical activity without a gym membership. If you work in an office, do you often email people that you could get up and go talk to around the corner? Do you interoffice mail a letter that you could walk and hand deliver? Take the stairs instead of the elevator at work to get calories burned and increase leg power and strength. Those are just some basic ideas to increase your daily physical activity.

Once you have started to incorporate simple types of physical activity, then look further into how you can cut down on your convenience transportation and utilize your own energy to get from one place to another. One of the best ways to incorporate physical activity into your life for minimal cost is to start bicycling to work. If your regular driving commute is during busy times of the day or you find yourself getting stopped by school buses on your way to work, you might actually be able to bike to work in the same amount of time as you could driving. Make sure you have a safe, well-fitting helmet and good reflection devices and clothing for your cycling trip. Check out appropriate clothing, helmets, and cycling gear at your local bike shop.

If your kids go to school close by and you are available to do so, start walking them to and from school instead of driving through traffic or putting them on the bus. By walking to school, you are increasing physical activity for you, but also for your children, which helps teach them to be physically active. Start to investigate grocery shopping that is within walking distance. Consider walking to destinations close to your home to get moving more.

Going to the gym and walking on a treadmill (going nowhere) is not going to help you lose weight more than walking outdoors. In fact, walking around your neighborhood might help you get to know your neighbors and allow you to have time out in nature.

If you often drive through the carwash, try washing your car by hand, which burns upwards of 200 calories. If you pay someone to do your home landscaping, save by mowing your own lawn, raking your own leaves, and pulling your own weeds. The idea is to consider what things decrease your physical activity and also cost you money. Substitute physical activity for items that you normally would depend on technology for and you will see an increase in your total daily caloric expenditure and money saved.

UNCONVENTIONAL EXERCISE

Perhaps the expense of a gym membership isn't as bothersome to you but the repetitious, traditional gym exercises are. It can feel monotonous to hit the gym every week and do the same machines and exercises. The hum of the treadmill and the music playing overhead in the weight room can feel like *Groundhog Day.*

If your brain is bored, chances are, your body is as well. Our bodies are wonderful at maintaining homeostasis, a constant state of biological equilibrium. Overtime, your once miserable cycling class can start to feel like a walk in the park. This can be due to your mental boredom as well as your physical boredom. Our bodies need constant overload to produce change. Overload is a term used for applying great loads to produce increased aerobic capacity or muscle tissue.

Without a change or increase in workout intensity, mode, frequency, or duration, your body hits a plateau. This plateau can feel miserable because you are putting out energy but not yielding results. Change it up to create some excitement in your workouts as well as elicit change in your body. If you are looking for things to do outside of the gym, then I suggest finding something you enjoy.

Rock climbing is an excellent workout. If you weigh 140 pounds, you can burn up to 700 calories an hour. I guarantee that is more than you would burn on an aerobic exercise machine for the same amount of time.

For anyone who likes dancing, Zumba is an extremely fun and challenging way to dance the calories off. Zumba can burn up to 600 calories per hour. Zumba is a combination of Latin, international, and cardiovascular dance. (You can buy a Zumba video at www.zumbasize.com.)

You can also take dance classes at a local dance studio. It is never too late to learn a new skill and dancing feels like a fun way to spend the evening, not like exercise. Plus, if you buy a dance video you can do it at home without feeling embarrassed.

Get outside to exercise. If you get outside, you will most likely encounter varying terrain or elevation when walking, running, or cycling. As you head out your front door you notice that the surface is not always even and your elevation can change, even if slightly. This will demand more of your balance and muscle coordination, which can carry over into other activities of daily living.

Grab a friend and explore a new hiking trail. You can even find groups to exercise with in the outdoors.

Walking videos can be very beneficial for those who want to be active but have with limitations that prevent them from getting outside of the house. You do burn slightly less calories walking or running in place than you do walking or running while moving. Yet a great benefit of walking in place is that you can do it anywhere, at any time. If the weather is too hot or too cold outdoors you can walk right in front of your television at home without the aid of any equipment. If you are traveling and do not have access to a gym or a safe place to be outside, then you can easily walk in place in your hotel room. Walking in place can prevent you from making any excuses not to stay active. And you can walk at any pace you want and not worry about changing terrain and elevation! The downside to walking in place is that it limits the muscles you are using as well as the dynamic coordination of your body. Our bodies are designed for moving from one place to another, therefore that is how our body responds best. Every time you take a step to propel your body forward, you are using many muscles and requiring slightly more energy (calories) to move your body as you push against the ground.

If a big reason for not exercising outside is your small children, and you really enjoy being outdoors, invest in a jogging stroller. You can purchase really nice double jogging strollers that will fit two large children and also increase your workout by helping you burn a lot more calories.

If you have older children, try to get outside with them and play a game of tag, touch football, or baseball. You will be surprised how much energy and agility is required of the sports you used to think were easy. Enjoy spending time with your kids while burning extra calories.

Don't underestimate how much living a healthy and active life can do for you. We often put exercise into a small box of lifting weights and hitting the treadmill. Yet being active is the objective. Just get your body moving! Most often, if you find an activity that you think is fun, you will want to do it more often and therefore, burn more calories. So get out there and enjoy trying something new!

WALKING THE DOG

Can man's best friend be a good exercise partner? As any pet owner knows, your furry friend needs exercise and that often involves you taking him out for a walk. Some studies have even found that dog owners get more physical activity time than those who are not dog-owners. This could be that your pet keeps you accountable because they enjoy the exercise so much. Here's how to make the most of your time with the pooch that will increase your physical fitness as well as theirs.

A dog can keep you going, but they can also be a distraction. Teaching your dog appropriate walking skills can help you get more walking time and less time smelling every bush and stopping for every other animal. Play catch or Frisbee with your pet pooch to get some extra activity.

How to walk your dog (from Judi James KPA-CTP from My Dogs Gym & Training Center):

1. Begin by marking and rewarding the dog for having a loose leash, then taking one step forward to mark and reward the dog for behaving and the leash staying loose.

2. Then take a step backward or sideways to again mark and reward the desired behavior.

3. Repeat this game about ten times.

4. Take a break and let the dog go and sniff or explore the grass or other interesting things around.

5. Then begin again at step one and increase the steps between each mark and reward. Once the dog is hanging around the handler's side waiting for the next reward, try going two steps forward and mark and reward for the leash being loose.

6. When the dog will stay with you for six or seven steps, try going longer distances between rewards.

7. Then try the same steps in different places with your dog.

Exercises to incorporate when walking your dog

- Before beginning, make sure that your dog sits during any of your stationary moves and learns to walk slowly next to you for any movement oriented exercises.

- **Lunge** – Maintain a slow gait while slowly incorporating walking lunges with the dog at your side.

- **Jog** – begin incorporating short bursts of jogging into your walk routine. This is good for you and your dog!

- **Bench pushups** – A park bench is a great tool for you to use. If your dog is well behaved you can keep the lead on your hand while doing ten pushups. If you need to, you can tie the lead to the bench while performing this and other bench exercises.

- **Bench step ups** – Either tie the dog to the bench or hold the lead tightly while you step up and down off a bench

- **Stair climbing** – Going up and down stairs is great workout for your legs and great for the dog's coordination and agility.

What to Buy:

- Front attachment harness, like the Wonder Walker Body Halter, to teach polite walking.

- Or a hip belt for the handler for hands free walking and running with your dog.

FITTING IN SIMPLE EXERCISES

If your days are jam-packed, it often feels impossible to fit in exercise. Yet if you have a non-stop schedule, finding time to exercise is vital for your health. There are a couple tips that will help you when trying to make time for exercise. First, remember that it takes moderate consistency to make a healthful impact. You do not need to go crazy in the gym seven days a week, just to end up losing weight and then quitting your gym membership. Lifelong health requires consistent, moderate exercise that is scheduled in a way that you can live with it for the long term!

Second, start to schedule your workouts in your calendar or day planner. You must put it in your calendar so other items such as meetings, dinner dates, and children's activities do not take over. If you sideline your health for too long, you will end up regretting it and find it much tougher to get started again. So schedule a moderate exercise plan that includes at least three days of moderate cardiovascular activity (light jog/brisk walking) and one or two days of resistance exercise. Even this reasonable amount will still make impactful change! You can probably fit in some stretching exercises in the evenings while kids are doing homework or the television is on.

Don't feel guilty for giving yourself the time to make healthy habits. If the weather is nice, have the family go out for a nice evening bike ride or walk after dinner. This allows for time to chat and helps model healthy behavior to everyone in the family.

If evenings are too busy, you can spread your cardiovascular activity throughout the day. Do ten or fifteen minutes of activity before work, then ten or fifteen minutes again on a lunch break, and more if you have time after work. Spreading your cardio time out might not help you shed the most pounds but it is good for your heart and still burns calories!

For resistance training, try these easy moves wherever you are (even on a quick break or while talking on the phone). Aim for twelve to fifteen of each:

- Pushups from your desk
- Squats
- Dips using your desk
- Isometric abdominal holds. While seated at your desk, pull your navel in toward your spine and contract your abs like someone is about to punch you in the stomach. Hold this for 20 seconds while breathing.
- Lunges

These flexibility exercises you can do anywhere:

- Seated hamstring stretch
- Seated hip flexor stretch
- Chest opening neck stretch

If your family is on the go, think outside the box:

- When your kids are at soccer/baseball practice: walk around the fields for exercise instead of sitting while watching.
- While standing and stirring dinner over the stove: squat into a heel raise for a quick toning move.
- If you live within walking distance to the store, try making one trip by foot. Or park the farthest away next time you are at the shopping mall or grocery store. All of those extra steps help!

different font size

SUMMER SPORTS AS EXERCISE

When the weather is warmer and dry, you can cover all of the basic components of an exercise program—while exercising outside! This includes cardiovascular exercise, resistance training, flexibility, and balance. It takes a few types of activities to incorporate the various components of a training plan, but you can easily do it all outdoors (or do some of it in the comfort of your home, if you prefer).

The best part about most outdoors sports is that they incorporate many of the components into one activity. Some of the best outside activities that burn a lot of calories are hiking, water skiing, and swimming. Roughly .037 calories are burned per minute, per pound during hiking. If you weigh 150 pounds and hike for sixty minutes, you will burn 333 calories. If you go for a day hike, you could burn many more calories. Make sure you pack plenty of liquids and nutritive foods if you are going to be hiking for a while. Make sure you go with someone else or at least tell people where you are going and when you plan to return.

Water skiing is fun way for the whole family to get physical activity in the summer. An hour of water skiing can burn 432 calories for a person who weighs 150 pounds. Water skiing can also build up a lot of upper body and core strength so this could be considered both cardiovascular and strength training.

Swimming is probably the most common way to get physical activity during the summer months. Many people swim year round in indoor pools, but pool use increases largely in the summer due to camps and outdoor pools opening. Swimming can burn 288 calories an hour for a person who weighs 150 pounds. Swimming is largely cardiovascular exercise and can greatly improve cardiorespiratory fitness.

To get in a full week of physical activity, it is recommended that you do cardiovascular exercise at least three, but preferably five to six days a week. If your family is planning to get on the boat and water ski on a Saturday or Sunday, you should try to get in a few more days of cardiovascular exercise in during the week. This could be a combination of swimming, hiking, jogging, or walking. Try to achieve at least twenty minutes of sustained cardiovascular exercise in any mode of your choice to get the full benefits. It is recommended that forty-five to sixty minutes of cardiovascular exercise be performed if you hope to lose weight.

To incorporate resistance training, here are a few different things to try. You can incorporate push-ups, lunges, and squats as part of your walk or jog. Or you could purchase a few hand weights and do at least two days of full body resistance training at home. You should try to do at least one set of twelve repetitions per muscle group, which should be about eight exercises.

For flexibility, be sure to stretch after each day of physical activity. If you cannot do it immediately where you are, it is a good idea to stretch before you fall asleep at night. This can be a nice calming way to finish up your day.

To incorporate balance and core strength, you can do planks, abdominal work, and one leg stork stands on your off day.

MAXIMIZING CALORIES BURNED

To maximize the total calories you burn in one workout, you should emphasize intensity over duration. That means you should focus on increasing your heart rate over the course of your workout. Both resistance training and cardiovascular training are important for weight loss and weight maintenance—as well as for heart health and muscular strengthening. To incorporate both resistance training and cardiovascular training, consider doing a circuit workout such as Tabata.

Tabata is a type of workout performed by completing a series of exercises back to back, at high intensity. A typical Tabata series includes at least six exercises that are each performed for twenty seconds back to back before taking thirty seconds to rest, and then repeating the series again. Complete this series eight times and it adds up to exactly twenty minutes of intense exercise. The great thing about the Tabata series is that you will be toning your muscles and increasing your heart rate. This will help increase your body's ability to work intensely while burning a lot of calories.

After a bout of intense Tabata circuit training, your body will have an increased level of excess post-exercise oxygen consumption (EPOC), which is the term for the elevated amount of oxygen your body consumes after a workout. If your body is consuming more oxygen, it means you are burning more calories. So a tough circuit workout will burn more calories post-workout then a slow jog might.

A great Tabata circuit includes the following exercises done in quick succession: sprinting, push-ups, sit-ups, shoulder lateral raises, squats, and dips. Perform each of the exercises for twenty seconds, moving quickly to the next one. Remember to have your space, weights, and equipment set up so that you do not take any rest between your six exercises until you have completed them all and are in your thirty second rest period. If you are new to resistance training or working out intensely then start by doing the exercises at your own pace or without any added weight.

I recommend doing the Tabata series two or three non-consecutive days of the week. Change the exercises that you are doing every few weeks so that your body does not get accustomed to the workout. If you can still manage to fit in regular weight training and cardiovascular workouts, your program will be well rounded and could increase your chances of continued success. Make sure that the exercises that you choose, when combined, provide an exercise for your entire body. You want a good blend of upper, lower, and core body exercises to get the best use of your time and energy.

Before starting a Tabata workout, get your body warmed up so that you do not have an injury. Walk in place or on a treadmill for about five minutes to warm up your muscles before working intensely. It can also help to set a timer on a watch to beep every ten seconds so that you can easily keep track of your time. If you find that you like this type of workout, you can create playlists on your MP3 player that plays music for 20 seconds and then pauses for 10 seconds to allow for a 10 second rest period. Programs to do this are available in Windows Media Player.

EXERCISE VIDEOS

Exercise videos have been around since Jane Fonda made them popular in the early 1980s. There are now tens of thousands of exercise videos for sale. So how can you choose which exercise video is appropriate, safe, and effective for you? After all, you can get an at-home workout video that focuses on weight loss, muscle building, strength training, dance, or yoga.

There is not one perfect video as everyone has different goals and physical history that will enable them to get different results. As well, different exercise video hosts motivate different people. The personality of hosts can make a big difference in whether you adhere to the video program or not. You can easily get referrals from friends and recommendations from magazines, view top sellers on shopping websites, or glean ideas from your personal trainer or doctor. Here are a few videos that offer a variety of workouts and techniques.

For the beginning yogi wanting weight loss: *Colleen Saidman's Yoga for Weight Loss* **by Gaiam**
This video offers three different twenty-minute segments that either provide a total body, abdominal focused, or strengthening and energizing workout. The movements are tailored to the beginner and are easily explained. You can perform just one of the twenty-minute sections or all three for a more intense workout. This is great for a beginner.

For the advanced yogi wanting an intense workout: *Bryan Kest's Power Yoga*
This video is more geared toward those who have some experience in yoga. There are three levels: beginner, intermediate, and advanced although most of the moves are actually advanced. To get an extreme workout, you can try for the advanced level and get an intense sweat-filled yoga session. The whole DVD is over two hours in length. As many of the moves are advanced, make sure you have physician approval, especially if you have had a history of back injury or pain.

Looking to dance your weight off: *Zumba Advanced*

If you can't make it to a Zumba class in person, try out this fun and calorie-burning dance session. The whole dance session is about forty minutes. This is a great way to torch calories and get your groove on. You won't even feel like you're exercising and the whole family could join in! Some of the steps can be a bit confusing if you haven't participated in a Zumba class before. For beginners, choose a more beginning level Zumba video.

For mind and body balance: *Intro to T'ai Chi* **by Gaiam**

T'ai Chi can offer a controlled way to improve balance, lower blood pressure, and provide mental clarity. This video offers three different segments: Entering the Flow for relaxation, Find the Still Point for more moves, and Create Balance for improving energy and coordination. Each segment lasts twenty minutes or you can do the whole DVD for sixty minutes. This is a great for any level or age group. The instructor is a highly decorated T'ai Chi master so you can be assured that your host is well qualified for teaching you.

For the most intense video out there: *Insanity*

You might have seen this video series on an infomercial. The series includes ten different videos that vary in focus from cardio to plyometric circuits. The duration of each video varies from thirty minutes to eighty-six minutes. This workout video series is only for those looking for an incredibly intense workout regimen. It is highly advisable to seek your physician's approval before starting this series. If you think at-home videos are too easy, this might be for you. Although the series is more expensive than others, it does offer ten videos that offer a large variety of workouts that can be done with your body weight.

CHAPTER 5

WEIGHT LOSS

Losing weight really has to do with a calorie deficit; you have to burn more calories than you eat. The average adult female might burn 1200-1500 calories a day doing very little to no physical activity. So if you are eating about that much and moving very little, you could still lose weight. Then again, you may not. You might be eating more calories than that, or your basal metabolic rate (calories burned at rest) might be less than the 1200-1500 calories/day. Some people who have very little muscle mass and are sedentary could have very low metabolic rates.

If your goal is to lose weight, then first make sure you are eating a diet full of healthy and nutritious foods. Many people who cut calories also cut out the nutrients in their diet. Try to aim for a diet full of plants (fruits, vegetables, legumes, and grains) so that you obtain the needed vitamins and minerals to have proper bodily functions and feel energetic. Also, eat frequently to keep your metabolism up since sever calorie restriction can slow your metabolism down. It is not suggested that adults eat below 1500 calories as this can cause a slowed metabolism. Below that range is not sufficient for sustainment of immune function amongst other necessary bodily functions.

Dieting might help you lose weight but it does not improve your fitness levels. The Aerobics Longitudinal Study found that men who were in the lowest quintile of fitness had a 3.13 times greater risk of dying from a stroke than those who were in the better fitness categories. Moving our bodies is essential to life. Flash back 200 years, and people were moving more. They had to forage for food, walk long distances, and work laboriously to survive. In our present society, where we have to move very little, we are gaining weight. We are becoming more diseased as well. Inactivity increases your risk for diabetes, heart disease, low back pain, and circulatory disorders. The Nurses Health Study found that walking two and a half hours or more a week decreased your risk for diabetes by 25 percent. The Harvard Alumni Study found that the relative risk of cardiovascular disease was 1.9 times greater for men who were inactive compared to those who spent their leisure time active.

Your body is meant to move! Inactivity can create joint and muscle stiffness, a lack of flexibility, and an increased risk of injury through daily activities. Exercise can increase your lean muscle mass and increase your metabolic rate, causing you to burn many more calories a day. As well, exercise has an emotional and mental effect. People who exercise have been found to have a better outlook on life and have a lower incidence of depression.

Exercise takes time but it could add years to your life. Physical activity is essential in maintaining bone and muscle health as well. Your bone mineral density drops quickly after the age of twenty. Exercise, especially resistance training, can increase muscle mass and by its pulling on the bone, can increase bone density as well. As well, exercise can decrease low back pain. Your vertebral discs need movement for fluid to move in and out of them properly. This will help you move more freely. Exercise can increase the strength of your low back and abdominal muscles. This will decrease your risk for low back injury; low back injury is the number reason for missed days at work in America.

So try combining healthy eating with exercise to get the best of both. You will lose weight and increase your fitness capabilities.

COMMUNITY SUPPORT

What makes some people adhere to their exercise goals and others not? A large amount of adherence could be predicted from the support they receive from their family and exercise partners. Researchers have found that people who receive support from their families or exercise group can largely affect their ability to adhere to their exercise program. Exercising with a group has many benefits and it might actually determine if you are successful or not. Although there are some people who are self-motivated to exercise, many others need external support and encouragement. Researchers from the Stanford Center for Research in Disease Prevention have shown in their studies to support the notion of external support in the form of exercising with others as a beneficial way to adhere to a program and stick with it over the long term.

Accountability

It is much too easy to hit the snooze button and go back to bed when no one is waiting for you at the gym or on the sidewalk for a morning jog. No one will know if you go back to bed, right? But eventually if you miss too many workouts, you will not receive the benefits persistence would bring. If you can find a partner or group to exercise with then you are more likely to stick to the program. Richard Pine, an avid group exerciser for the past seventeen years, says, "When I could go and exercise on my own time, I never did it. But when I made appointments with a group exercise class, I did it. I followed through." He says group exercise works for him because it has a distinct start and ending time.

A great strategy for group accountability is creating a network with others who have similar goals. One idea is have a group reward only if everyone meets a target. For example, get four of your friends together and each set a goal (e.g., exercising two times/week). Once you complete your exercise, text or email the rest of the group to keep track. Everyone can have different individual goals but if not everyone meets their individual goal, and then no one in the group receives the reward. Maybe the reward after a month of hitting all targets is going out for an after work dinner, appetizer, or massage! If one person doesn't reach their goal, then the whole group doesn't get the reward. This keeps everyone accountable.

Motivation

A group exercise class, group run, or cycle ride can be a great way to increase your workout intensity. We tend to amp up our intensity when amongst others. Pine says, "Stealing energy from the instructor and classmates" keeps him inspired to work harder. If you are accustomed to going for a jog alone but find you are skipping workouts or taking it easy, find a partner or group to go out and run with. Your pace will often be pushed and you will feel motivated to keep up. One group runner, Ann Hill, says, "I look forward to my Saturday morning group runs, because I couldn't endure those long miles alone." If you enjoy exercise classes, find someone in the class you want to keep up with. Challenge yourself to work your hardest and enjoy being pushed by others.

Social Aspects

Most people love to build relationships with others and it can be fun, rewarding, and exciting to meet new people with a common goal. Ann Hill says, "The friendships that I've established mean the world to me. Getting together to run helps me achieve my running goals and share those successes with others who have this common interest."

Many seniors tend to adhere to exercise because of the social interactions involved with their activity. For example, many retirement homes, athletic clubs, and therapy clinics offer group classes and find that the participants develop friendships that extend beyond the workout time. In fact, research has shown that people who have a social network tend to live longer and happier lives. So not only will group exercise benefit your physical self, it can also nurture your emotional and psychological health. If you are looking to increase your activity level, seek out a group to do it with.

5 Tips to staying accountable in a group:

1. Set a time in your calendar for an exercise class.
2. Meet with a friend at least once a week for a workout.
3. Join an accountability group that rewards only when everyone succeeds.
4. Schedule a group workout during a normally stressful time in the day. It will encourage you!
5. Tell a friend. It is helpful to tell others what your goals are; you'll be more likely to achieve them if everyone knows!

EXERCISING FOR WEIGHT LOSS

If you are exercising to lose weight, the length of time you exercise is completely dependent upon how much weight you want to lose, how accustomed to exercise your body is, and how many calories you eat on a daily basis. For the average, healthy weight American, the Surgeon General recommends thirty to sixty minutes of physical activity every day. That is more than most Americans get daily!

If your goal is weight loss, then the Surgeon General suggests up to ninety minutes a day, as does the American College of Sports Medicine. However, if you are new to exercising, this will feel like a physical hardship and impossible to fit into your busy schedule. So I suggest you work your way up to the sixty to ninety minutes by slowly incorporating daily physical activity in twenty or thirty minute increments.

What kind of exercise should you perform for weight loss? If you are not accustomed to exercise, you should start slow and work up. You could perform a few ten minute segments, multiple times in a day, to get as much movement as you can.

If you are already accustomed to thirty minutes of activity at a time, then I suggest you do two things: increase the length of activity and the intensity. Where most people go wrong is their intensity. They often think that a leisure walk on the treadmill will help them lose fat. Although that's better than nothing, more and more research shows that higher intensity exercise will burn that fat quicker. Why? Higher intensity exercise increases your heart rate and total caloric burn—that means many more calories burned!

To incorporate high intensity moves on a treadmill or bicycle, try adding sprinting for thirty seconds every two minutes. This is called interval training. If you tend not to push yourself hard enough, opt for a higher intensity group exercise class such as spinning, kickboxing, or other intense workouts. That way your instructor can push you past your comfort zone, which is most likely necessary if you want to make some major physical changes.

The length of your workouts might depend on how
much you eat or how much weight you want to lose. But first ~space
know that you should never justify eating more because you
had a good workout. This usually causes your hard work to
backfire because you will most likely eat more calories than
you burned at the gym, therefore sabotaging your entire
sweat-busting workout!

Losing fat is a math game. You have to burn more
calories than you eat to lose weight. We often overestimate
how many calories we burn at the gym and underestimate
how many calories we eat. That ends up costing us on the
scale. Try food logging to see an accurate picture of your
caloric intake. Log your workouts with it; this will help you
figure out how you are equalizing your workouts to your
energy intake. If you aren't sure how many calories you are
burning during a workout, you might want to invest in a heart
rate monitor watch that will track calories burned. Watches like
this, made by Polar and Mio, Nike, and Apple will determine
your caloric burn based on your heart rate and body weight
and can be a more accurate way to log workout progress. In
fact, such watches can tell you if you are improving physically
by showing a lower heart rate at the same exercise intensity.

To lose weight, it might be wise to increase the length
of your workouts but be realistic. We all only have so many
hours in the day. If you run out of time, amp up the intensity!

Intense workouts will help you burn more calories and build lean muscle, which will make you stronger and healthier!

LOSING WEIGHT FOR AN EVENT

If a wedding, reunion, or another special event is quickly approaching, you may be inspired to step up your exercise to lose weight and look your best. What's the best method? Should you focus your time on doing cardio to burn calories or weight train to gain some muscle tone?

Cardiovascular exercise is absolutely essential for heart health and overall respiratory endurance but might not be your ticket to a toned, sleek body for your event. I have seen many people spend countless minutes, even hours, on the elliptical machine or walking on the treadmill trying to achieve some magical calorie burn. Although this type of exercise has its time and place in everyone's program, it is not going to help you torch calories and therefore lose weight. The old myth that doing cardio at a lower target heart rate (shown as the fat-burning zone on most cardio machines) will burn more calories from fat is confusing. Although exercising at a lower heart rate will burn a larger percentage of calories from fat, you will burn far fewer calories overall when you are exercising at a lower intensity. If you can increase your intensity (by increasing speed, incline, or resistance), you will have a higher total caloric burn. And its total calories burned and caloric deficits that will help you lose weight!

Instead of sauntering on the treadmill while watching your favorite soap opera, amp up your intensity. I suggest that you combine both high intensity circuits (like weight training) with interval cardio workouts through your week. On Monday, Wednesday, and Friday perform a full body circuit weight training program. An example would be to do the following exercises over and over, each for thirty seconds: Jump rope, squats, push-ups, lunges, two arm dumbbell bent rows, squat jumps, and then sit ups. Repeat this circuit over and over again for twenty to thirty minutes with a one-minute rest break in the middle. On Tuesday and Thursday, perform twenty to thirty minutes of interval training doing your favorite cardio exercise. If you like the treadmill, then alternate thirty seconds of sprinting with one minute of jogging (beginning with a five-minute warm-up and ending with a five-minute cool-down). If you enjoy the elliptical, then increase the intensity for at least thirty seconds at a time but maintain your RPMs. If you are up for trying a new cardio workout, go for the Stairmaster, jump rope, or do plyometrics (e.g., jumping up and down off a box). Any type of exercise that will increase your heart rate will burn more calories. If you want to, take a lower-intensity walk or jog on Saturday. Then rest on Sunday to recover.

Remember, if your total goal is weight loss and increased tone, you will have to eat wisely as well. Make sure you eat a healthy and balanced breakfast, lunch, and dinner. If you need a snack in between, then grab fruits and vegetables instead of pre-packaged snacks. The more natural your food, the more energy you will have for working out. In fact, make sure you are supplying your body with enough calories to workout hard. Many people eat too little and then try to hit the gym. This will cause you to work less intensely and burn fewer calories, so feed your body complex carbohydrates, lean proteins, and healthy fats.

Be kind to yourself. It is not wise to lose weight too fast. It took time to gain it, and you should not lose more than one or two pounds a week for long term success. Resist the urge to weigh yourself daily. Instead weigh yourself every Saturday morning and log this so you can go back and see how you are doing. It might also be a good idea to have a certified trainer measure your body fat so you know if you are losing muscle. If you lose muscle while losing weight, your overall metabolism will slow, causing a slowed weight loss.

DIETING WITHOUT STARVING

Dieting can feel like the most frustrating thing in the world. The hardest part is cutting calories without feeling like you're starving. It's difficult to convince your body that you don't really need that pint of ice cream every night while watching your favorite show.

There are a few things happening in your body when you start cutting calories. The first problem is the physical fixation with eating and snacking. Most of us can do fairly well eating a healthy breakfast and lunch and then we slowly lose willpower as the day goes on. By late afternoon, we are ravenous and snack before dinner, eat dinner, and then keep snacking until bedtime. You can easily get into a physical routine of having something in your mouth to chew on while sitting in front of the television. So in a sense, this is a food addiction. Compare this to a cigarette smoker who is comforted and addicted to holding the cigarette as much as they are with the nicotine.

Added to the physical addiction to munching is the physical hunger. You might very well be hungry if your body is used to a higher intake of calories from day to day. If you suddenly drop the calories you are eating, then your body will fight that starvation feeling with hunger and a slowed metabolism. Your stomach is most likely enlarged to fill the food that you normally fill it with. So less food might not actually fill your stomach like extra servings and large portions did. But it is possible to change from eating way too much to eating less in order lose weight—without starving!

There are a few tricks you can use to trick your body into losing weight and not slowing its metabolism. If you drop calories too fast and too drastic, you will have a slowed metabolism and over time, even lower calories will not allow you to lose weight. So you have to trick your body's natural reaction to starvation.

First, eat a large breakfast even if you aren't hungry. You might not feel hungry for breakfast if you are not used to eating a nutritious breakfast. Start your day with a large breakfast made of complex carbohydrates (such as old fashioned oats), protein (such as eggs/egg whites), and a small amount of fat to keep you satisfied (such as peanut butter). Next, have a nutritious snack three hours after you eat breakfast! Do not miss this little snack as it will signal to your brain that you are not starving. A small snack should be an apple with a small amount of almond butter, or cottage cheese and strawberries, or two cups air popped popcorn with a cheese stick.

Eat a lunch that fills up that room in your stomach. Eat a lot of roughage (green vegetables, like a salad) to make you feel full but provide few calories. On top of the salad add a lean protein like chicken, and a healthy olive oil and vinegar dressing; pile on as many colorful vegetables as you can! Fiber helps you feel fuller and satiated. Also, make sure you are eating enough fat. You should eat 20-30 percent of your daily calories from fat—but from healthy sources like seeds, nuts, and plant oils.

Have a mid-afternoon snack like you did in the morning and eat a nutritious dinner. Dinner should be centered on your vegetables, whole grain rice or red potato, and a lean protein. Again, make sure there is some fat there. And if you are hungry in the evening, have a portion-controlled snack and drink lots of water to fill you up.

These tips will give you the nutrition you need to lose weight without feeling like you're starving: eat breakfast, eat small portions often, drinks lots of water, and don't avoid fat as it will help you feel full and satisfied. It is impossible to always accurately count calories so if you are hungry, grab a healthy option. If you always reach for a fruit or vegetable first, you will most likely cut out processed foods that were contributing to your weight loss plateau.

DIET SODA

You might have heard it on the news or read it in the paper, but the news is traveling fast. Research now claims that drinking diet soda will cause weight gain. How can something without calories cause you to gain weight?

The University of Texas Health Science Center studied 1,550 men and women to see diet soda's effect on weight.

They found that 57 percent of those who drank two or more cans of diet soda a day became overweight after eight years. This is compared to the 47 percent from the control group who drank regular drinks. What does this mean and how can this occur? The answer isn't in the calories you are drinking but in how that drink might affect your body.

When you drink a lot of diet soda your body receives no nutritional density (a sense of fullness or satisfaction). Diet soda drinkers tend to rationalize that they are saving a lot of calories by avoiding regular soda and therefore end up eating more than the regular soda drinkers do. It is this mentality that causes many people to drink diet soda with several slices of pizza. If you use diet soda as a means to rationalize eating more calories then you are sabotaging your diet hopes.

Another theory lies in the effect on metabolism when diet soda is used as a food substitute. If you feel hungry but drink a diet coke instead of eating, you send your brain mixed signals. Your body recognizes you are ingesting liquids but you are not providing your body with any nutrients. When you finally eat hours later, your metabolism is slower because you haven't eaten food with nutrients and calories.

The Framingham Heart Study followed over 9,000 men and women, and shows that consuming diet soda is related to metabolic syndrome, which is a collection of risk factors such as cardiovascular disease, diabetes, abdominal obesity, high cholesterol, abnormal blood sugar levels, and high blood pressure.

So should you drink diet soda? And is diet soda better for you than regular soda since regular soda has so much sugar in it? It depends on how much you drink and your other dietary intake. If you are limiting yourself to one or fewer cans of diet soda a day then research shows that it will not terribly harm you. Take into consideration that you are ingesting artificial sweeteners; there is a lot of controversy regarding the safety of artificial sweeteners. Eat something light with your diet soda for your metabolism. Remember, drinking diet soda does not allow you to eat more calories.

Regular soda does contain high amounts of sugar. A twelve-ounce can of soda can have as much as thirteen teaspoons of sugar in the form of high fructose corn syrup. High fructose corn syrup has been shown to alter the function of your metabolism and has addictive properties. So try to avoid or limit your ingestion of regular soda as well.

The best liquid you can drink is good, plain water. Water is the most pure form of liquid. Your body needs water for every bodily function. If you are thirsty, your body probably needs water and not regular or diet soda.

Limit your intake of both regular soda and diet soda since regular soda contains a lot of sugar and diet soda has been shown to increase your body weight.

AVOIDING WEIGHT GAIN WHEN QUITTING SMOKING

If you are worried that quitting smoking will cause you to gain weight, consider what you are eating. Remember that smoking may have taken up much of your spare time before. Smoking often keeps your hands and mouth busy and can sidetrack you from eating. If you take the cigarettes away, you might discover the desire to eat more with your spare time. As well, the desire to snack more could possibly be caused by a decrease in serotonin levels after you quit smoking. Eating carbohydrates and fatty rich meals would cause your serotonin levels to increase and make you feel better. But you don't have to handle it that way. These hormone levels will adjust back to normal eventually.

If you feel increased cravings, make sure to have healthy snacks on hand such as whole-wheat pretzels, all natural peanut butter, and fresh fruit. Try to reach for healthy, portion-controlled snacks when the urge arises and you need something to eat.

FRUIT SUGARS AND BODY FAT

There are so many different tips and ideas on what to eliminate and how to best lose body fat. According to the 2009 Center for Disease Control Report on Fruits and Vegetables, only 33 percent of adults are getting enough fruits and only 27 percent are getting enough vegetables. And there has been an increasing push to increase American consumption of fruits and vegetables. Why? Fruits and vegetables have been found to reduce the risk of some types of cancers, lower the risk for heart disease, diabetes, and promote growth and cell repair in children and adults.

So does cutting out fruits help you lose body fat? That all depends on a few factors. If you were the type of person who normally consumes a large amount of fruits and suddenly cut them out, you could have a reduction in caloric intake which could help you lose weight. But what if you substitute the fruit intake with other sweet foods that might not be healthy for you?

Our bodies are hard-wired to desire the naturally occurring sweet taste found in fruits. What can often happen if you are not getting the sweet-fix from naturally occurring sugars in fruit is that you will go after other, manufactured sweets. If you reach for processed sweets such as soda and desserts, you will be worse off.

So why does cutting fruit out help some people lose weight? This again can be from a caloric deficit, but much if it can also be the loss of water. Much of fruit is water and is often a large source of total body water for most people. If you are not eating fruits or starchy vegetables (a common diet practice), you will be cutting out much of the water you normally get in food.

Some fitness experts say that cutting out fruit will, in time, shut off that sweet tooth desire completely. There is a slight bit of truth to this. Sweetness is addictive. Your body wants more of those sweet tasting foods so that you can store the glucose for future energy needs. But this desire can backfire if you eat something sweet and continue on eating something sweet until you are stuffed and you have eaten too many sugars.

If you are eating lots of fruit without complementary proteins and healthy fats, this can cause an increase in blood sugar and then a quick drop as sugars found in fruit can be quickly digested and hit the blood stream rapidly. So if you eat a banana or apple without anything with it, you could end up wanting more and more in the very near future.

Cutting out fruit is not necessary. You should continue to eat the recommended three to five servings of each fruits and vegetables daily to ensure that you are obtaining crucial vitamins and minerals such as Vitamin C, folate, magnesium, and potassium. Eat the fruit with a healthy fat such as peanut butter or a lean meat such as chicken. This will help slow down the digestive process of the meal. That means a lower spike in blood glucose and slower drop in blood glucose as well. This will prevent you from the continuing desire to eat more and more.

For some people, it helps them to consume most of their fruits early in the day so that their body can burn the glucose. Then they eat the majority of their vegetables later in the day. Try this to see if you notice any major changes. Always remember that it is never a good practice to cut out entire food groups that are good for you. Diets that require you to cut out healthy foods will often help you lose weight initially either from water loss or calorie deficit, but the results are short lived. Your body needs a well-balanced diet that supplies the nutrients your body needs to maintain enzymatic and immune function. Eat a diet that is rich in natural foods and stay away from processed items and you will be healthier!

SPLURGING ON FUN FOOD

Even if you've eaten well all week and only splurge on one Saturday night pig-out, you will probably have to pay hard for that one big night out.

Let me give you just a few examples of a typical meal out and the amount of calories you would need to burn off that meal. Some menu items might shock you a little! I am not at all against any of these restaurants; in fact, I most likely have eaten there or else I would not know or care about the contents of their menu!

The first place is Red Robin, which is such a fun place to go and celebrate with friends and family. The obvious guilty pleasure is a cheeseburger. Their guacamole bacon burger has 1156 calories and 77 grams of fat. You would have to jog at five mph for 100 minutes to burn that off. If you add an order of onion rings (adds 1251 calories and 65 grams of fat) then you have to do an additional 108 minutes. So that is a total of 208 minutes or three and a half hours of jogging at five mph! And this is without any beverages! A surprising order that puts you back on the treadmill is the crispy chicken tender salad, which packs 1325 calories and 83 grams of fat. Again that is almost two hours of jogging at five mph!

Another common treat is pizza. A typical slice of pepperoni pizza has 370 calories and 18 grams of fat. You can save about a hundred calories per slice if you order thin crust. If you eat two slices of pepperoni pizza, you would need to swim for two and a half hours to burn that off! I think that we all know pizza is a guilty pleasure, but it is a common choice.

What about those giant steaks—similar to the ones you can eat and then get free if you finish it? A porterhouse steak at Outback Steakhouse will portion you 1230 calories and 99 grams of fat. If you add the Bloomin' Onion (which has 2310 calories and 134 grams of fat), you are asking for about five or six hours of yard work or a walk at four pmh for 580 minutes—

almost six hours! Personally, I am not sure if those morsels are worth that much exercise!

One last pig out weekend favorite is ice cream. Who doesn't love going out to ice cream with the kids on a Saturday night? Most of the Cold Stone Creamery Gotta Have It sizes of ice cream have around 340 calories. This is not where we go wrong. It is the mix-ins. If you add in brownies (for 170 calories), caramel (90 calories), and pecan pralines (240 calories), you are now at 840 calories. And if you put that in a waffle dipped cone you are adding another 310 calories for a grand total of 1150 calories. To burn that guilty pleasure off, you will need to do water aerobics for about three hours. Remember that Cold Stone offers many healthier options such as all fruit sorbet and sinless ice creams without the fat.

None of this means you can never enjoy your food or indulge in tasty treats. However, you should be aware that it takes a 3500 calorie deficit to lose a pound. Let's imagine you are really good for most of the week, eating about 500 calories below your maintenance calories each day, Monday through Friday. If you do this, you might be at a 2500 calorie deficit by Friday night. But if you go out on Saturday night and eat around 3500 calories for dinner and dessert in just one night, then you do not have a total deficit for that week at all. In fact, you just ruined all the hard work you did during the week.

So instead, go out with your friends and share a menu item with a friend. I think sharing is better than doggy bagging and taking it home, which only allows you to eat the unhealthy food for another meal. Just share it or order a small portion of an appetizer that will satisfy you just as well. This will save you many calories!

Learn to enjoy your food. Enjoy every bite, without devouring it. I also suggest not drinking any alcohol as that is additional calories and alcohol tends to inhibit your sense of satiety. You will eat more when you drink! Instead drink water, which will help fill you up and hydrate you.

AVOIDING WEIGHT GAIN AT THE HOLIDAYS

If you are being careful about eating, it can feel like you are the only one at a holiday gathering that eats healthy; that everyone notices if you do not fill your plate with butter-laden fare. You could very well be the only person in the crowd that is trying to watch the calories going in your mouth or it might be that everyone else feels the same way you do and no one is talking about it. Holiday gatherings at work or with family and friends can feel like a high-pressure situation to let your guard down and lose any self-control over high calorie foods and drinks. But no one else at the party has to live with the pounds you gain from eating too much food! So what do you do to save your body and still enjoy the party? I have a few suggestions.

Eat a small meal within three hours of the party to make sure you aren't ravenous when all that tempting food stares you down. Make the meal light, with a lean protein, fibrous whole grains, and a small portion of healthy fat to help fill you up.

Also, hydrate the day of a big party. Being hydrated will help you feel fuller and will help prevent dehydration that happens with drinking alcohol. On the day of a big event, stick to your regular exercise routine to help burn calories and keep your metabolism up. This all may be fairly easy to manage but what happens when you show up at the party? What can you eat and what shouldn't you?

In the December 2010 issue of Women's Health Magazine, there was a great article by Karen Ansel, R.D. about what foods to eat and which ones to stay away from at your holiday party. Here are some of the best food options that were given in the article: instead of the mini-crab cakes that can have 170 calories and 11 grams of fat, opt for the bacon wrapped scallops that have around 110 calories and 3.6 grams of fat. Instead of a handful of mixed nuts that can pack 219 calories and 20 grams of fat, choose ten large olives, which have 51 calories and 5 grams of fat.

When it comes to drinks, choose champagne over champagne or cocktail mixers. A six-ounce glass of champagne has 130 calories. Other dangerously high caloric drinks are eggnog, brandy alexanders, and blended drinks like margaritas and coladas. A cup of regular eggnog has 340 calories and 14 grams of fat, which is mostly saturated. Eight ounces of brandy alexander has 683 calories and 22 grams of fat. Talk about packing a punch on your daily caloric tally! The average margarita has close to 350 calories and a mixed drink made with rum (like a piña colada) has at least 300 calories. Lower calorie options include a wine spritzer (around 70 calories) or a five-ounce glass of white wine (about 120 calories).

The most important things to remember are to enjoy both the food and the socializing. If you are going to take something to eat or drink, then enjoy it. That often means sitting down with your food and tasting every bite instead of eating while you are talking. Talking causes you to miss how good the food tastes as well as to be distracted from the conversation. Try to sip your drink and follow each beverage with a large glass of water. This will help fill you up and lower the amount of high calorie drinks you consume. Limit yourself to one time around the buffet table and grab the items that are most appealing. Leave the items that do not interest you and try not to return to the food table. Enjoy the atmosphere; get out on the dance floor and dance with your friends or just enjoy meeting new people and the conversation.

Beyond parties, holiday meals can be extremely challenging to even consider thinking about how many calories you are eating. Should you just forget healthy eating for Thanksgiving and the days that follow! After all, it's also hard to exercise on Thanksgiving Day or the entire weekend when it is full of shopping! I understand the approach of taking the weekend a little lax and letting loose. However, be aware that the average Thanksgiving dinner can rack up to over 3,000 calories! Now these 3,000 calories are just Thanksgiving dinner, not the mindless munching all afternoon that leads to dinner and the Friday and Saturday of leftovers.

A little mathematic reminder: 3,500 calories equals a pound. If you eat an extra 3,500 calories, you will gain a pound. In just your Thanksgiving dinner, you have the chance of putting on a pound of fat that will stay with you. If you continue to overeat throughout the weekend, you can increase the pounds you will gain.

This might all sound very depressing and could reinforce your "forget about it" mentality. Try to not think of it as all or nothing. Take little steps that might help your chances of your jeans fitting come New Year's Day. Although many health clubs are closed on Thanksgiving and Christmas, you can get outside, rain or shine, for a jog/walk or a fun flag football game with the family. Any type of activity will increase your calorie expenditure which can help prevent all those calories of holiday food from adding up to increased body weight. Move any way you can on a big eating holiday.

When it comes to eating on Thanksgiving Day, try to eat in a normal pattern leading up to the meal. Instead of thinking that you will starve all day to deserve a large meal later, eat your regular breakfast, healthy mid-morning snack, and lunch. This will prevent you from over-eating at dinner and keep your metabolism revved up to take on that heavy Thanksgiving dinner. When you arrive at your Thanksgiving meal destination and all the appetizers and snack foods are staring you in the eye, try to do these three things. First, pick the healthier options such as fruits and vegetables (sans a lot of dip) and even high fiber hummus. Then stop at one small plate. Second, drink a lot of water leading up to the meal to stay hydrated which will aid in digestion and also prevent you from over-eating. Third, when dinner is served, be choosey. Choose only the foods that you actually like. Do not waste an extra 400 calories on green bean casserole if it's not your favorite. If you are going to indulge, you should indulge in food that you enjoy and tastes good, not just because it is there and being served.

If you know you love your aunt's pecan pie, then eat your dinner with that in mind. Eat slowly and enjoy each bite.

Take at least fifteen to thirty minutes to let your brain realize how much you ate before digging in to dessert. You can still eat a healthy portion of turkey and sweet potatoes, but remember that the slice of pecan pie will give you an extra 450 calories.

You can have that piece of pie, but do you really need a piece that is a quarter of the pie? Take a smaller portion, sit down, and enjoy every bite. When you are done with that piece, wait fifteen minutes and see if you are still hungry before taking any more. If you eat too fast, then your brain cannot keep up and you will not realize how full you are, while continuing to eat.

In the days that follow Thanksgiving, many people are busy shopping in crowded malls, eating leftovers, and grabbing food on the go. If you know you are hitting the malls, then pack an apple, some almonds, and a healthy protein bar. Go prepared. Most people go either way on Thanksgiving weekend. They either get tons of sleep while relaxing and eating too much food, or they go like mad trying to get ready for Christmas and so lose sleep and time to exercise. Neither option is very healthy. Try to get a good night's sleep so you do not mistake hunger for lack of sleep. And if you are eating leftovers and lying around the house, eat adequate portions and get your exercise. In fact, invite the family over to help you eat all the extra food!

Enjoy every moment of the holidays and being with your loved ones without the entire focus being on food. Eat your meals slowly and enjoy the conversation and maintain an active lifestyle throughout the hectic weekend and you won't find yourself fighting the holiday pounds later.

AVOIDING WEIGHT GAIN ON VACATION

When you're on track with diet and exercise, you don't want a vacation to ruin all of your hard work. If you do not exercise at all on a vacation, you will not likely lose any strength, but you will likely gain weight, especially since what you eat while you are vacationing can sabotage your body just as much as the lack of activity!

Yet you can easily enjoy your vacation without indulging at every meal. If you really want that ice cream cone, then go for a kid size scoop and enjoy every bite. You can still enjoy food without eating until you are sick! If the location that you are going to is new or you aren't sure what your grocery options will be, pack some healthy foods. You can carry individual packets of oatmeal for breakfast, protein or granola bars for snacking, raw almonds, dried fruit, and even protein powder in your suitcase. Often foreign countries offer great beaches and swimming pools but questionable sources of food. So supply yourself with food you know is healthy and safe.

Make sure the hotel you are staying in has a fitness center of some kind. It is much easier to exercise if it is in the same building as you. If your spouse takes the kids to the pool or if your family tends to sleep in later than you do, you can take advantage of this time for yourself and hit the gym. A great website is www.whenwetravel.com. They list hotels that have fitness centers so you can search for hotels specifically this way. They list hotels all over the world. There are other sites such as www.hotels.com that will give you fitness centers as a search parameter as well.

If you are dead set on a hotel because of its location or other amenities but it does not have a fitness center, then you can easily find area fitness centers. In your web browser, put in your destination and "fitness center/gym" and it will give you all area options. I always opt for a location that I can walk or jog to so I can get extra exercise and avoid the drive.

Oftentimes, going to a gym while you are at a beautiful locale can be depressing and daunting. Remember that vacations can be active! Schedule a family hike or snorkeling tour. You will get a day full of exercise and hardly realize you are burning all those calories. Many places that you visit are beautiful and offer many stunning views that are best seen while hiking or swimming. If you are in an unfamiliar place, make sure to hire a reputable guide to ensure your safety.

Try to fit exercise into the daily lifestyle of your vacation. If your hotel does not have a fitness center and the area is not safe for a jog, then try to take a stroll up and down the beach while the kids make sand castles. Many trips can offer tours and adventures that your family will remember and your body will be grateful for.

Just in case you can find no options and your family would rather lounge poolside, pack these exercise essentials:

- Exercise band/tubing with handles
- Jump rope
- Deflated exercise ball

You can usually sneak in twenty minutes a day to do an in-room workout with these three essentials. If your hotel cannot assist you in blowing up your ball, a local gas station is sure to have an air hose for tires and you can use this to inflate your exercise ball.

Here is a basic workout: start with three minutes of jumping rope to warm up. Do two minutes of stretching and then three minutes of core crunches on the ball and thirty seconds of planks. Then use your exercise tube for resistance while you squat and also for overhead presses, side raises, bicep curls, and triceps extensions.

You might not lose more weight or gain much muscle while vacationing, but you can definitely maintain your fitness level. Then when you return home, you will not have any "vacation weight" to lose or muscle toning to catch up on. You will look as good as new when you return!

LOSING LOWER BODY FAT

For most women, the thighs are the toughest area to get lean and lose body fat. Women tend to carry more subcutaneous (right under the skin) fat in their thighs, hips, and buttocks then men do. This is common for most women and cannot be avoided for many. However, overall body fat and lean muscle mass will affect how much fat you carry. What areas you carry the fat is not necessarily decided or controlled by you. Genetics plays a huge role.

There are a few mistakes that many people make when trying to lose fat in areas such as their thighs. The first problem could be over-working your legs. Not allowing for enough recovery time or doing too much of the same exercises can reduce the chances of losing the leg fat. Exercises need to vary to ensure that you work all of the muscles. Forget doing just leg extensions, leg curls, and hip extensions. You need to start performing multiple-joint movements such as squats, lunges, and step ups to increase the caloric burn and work all of the muscles of the leg. Resistance training can be performed with your legs two days a week, spread out by a few days of rest in between. Make sure that those two days are intense; complete three sets of twelve to fifteen repetitions of at least three to four exercises. On your other days, work your upper body and incorporate cardiovascular exercise. Vary the type of cardio you perform with jogging, walking, swimming, biking, or other forms of cardio.

A great way to shed extra body fat off of your lower body is through plyometric training. Plyometric training—jump training—will increase the intensity of your workout. The intense nature of plyometrics and muscular and cardiovascular demand will help shed some extra fat. Start by doing simple plyometrics by adding jump squats or jump split lunges to your lower body weights days. Once you have mastered those two, try jumping up onto a box and down. Aim for a completion of time, such as thirty seconds, or for repetitions, such as twelve. Make sure you give your legs plenty of rest time in between plyometric training.

Nutrition is a key to losing overall body fat. Ironically, people trying to lose weight will often restrict calories too much. If you cut back on your dietary intake too much, you will lose muscle as much as fat and this can cause a reduction in the appearance of muscle tone. You could lose weight with calorie restriction but the overall leanness of your legs might suffer. A diet that reduces body fat includes lots of leafy green vegetables, low glycemic fruits such as berries, and lean meats and fish. Eat a fairly planned diet day to day and allow yourself more flexibility on Saturday or Sunday. Eat three meals a day with two or three snacks in between—all focused on healthy nutrition. You also must stay hydrated. Skin that is well hydrated will have a better appearance. Plus, dehydration often causes people to overeat.

If in doubt, move more and improve the quality of dietary intake. Be patient with your body because your genetic make-up has much to do with where your body carries fat and where you lose it first. Do the best you can by eating a nutritious diet and keep a varied exercise plan.

LOSING ARM FAT

As with losing leg fat, it is good to remember that there is no such thing as spot reduction; but there might be something such as spot muscle toning. If you want your arms to be more toned, then you need to work your arms. However, it is true that you cannot do arm curls and triceps dips in hopes to see chiseled arms without any fat to cover them up. You will have to amp up your entire workout routine to see a real improvement in your arms and your waistline. The reason is that your body will gain and lose weight in the places that it wants to.

You could have well-toned arms hiding underneath subcutaneous fat. If that is the case, then you will need a good dose of cardiovascular training, strength training, and a healthy eating plan.

To get started, you will have to increase what you are already accomplishing. If you are a regular exerciser and go to the gym a few times a week, then you are on the right track. You will most likely just need an updated workout plan. Are you finding that your cardio routine is the same each time? Do you get on the elliptical machine and coast while watching your favorite television show? If so, then you might want to try something new. Try out a new cardio class such as Zumba, kickboxing, or spinning. The group and intensity will increase your motivation and caloric burn.

If you are not currently exercising, add a few days of a walk-jog interval workout. Start with twenty minutes: warm up for three minutes, then do a one minute jog with a one minute walk, alternating to complete your time. Once this is easy, lower your walk breaks and increase your total time. If you can hit the gym, try a weight training class so you can learn good form and make sure to hit all of the important muscle areas. If you have time afterward, do a few extra arm exercises to ensure you are covered.

If you are not a member of a gym, invest in a couple pairs of dumbbells you can use at home. You will want them to be heavy enough that a set of ten bicep curls is challenging (try ten in the store before you purchase). Do this weight training circuit three times a week: pushups, lunges, overhead press, bicep curls, jump squats, overhead triceps extensions, and then side lateral raises. Once you have completed one set of twelve repetitions of each, rest for two minutes and repeat the entire circuit one or two more times.

One of the most basic exercises that can improve your arms is the push-up. Push-ups are not always easy but they help increase muscle strength and toning in your triceps, the back of your arms, and your chest. If traditional push-ups are difficult, then try to do them with your hands elevated on a bench or with your knees on the ground. Focus on a full range of motion to increase functional length but also the length of your arm muscles.

The shoulder muscles are incredibly important for visual appeal of the arms since they give the arms tone and shape. The deltoid muscles attach about a third of the way down the side of your upper arm (your humerus bone). Bringing your arms directly to the side of your body, called abduction, strengthens the deltoid muscles and can improve the shape of your arms. A good exercise for toning the deltoid muscles are lifting your arms out to the sides, called a lateral raise, with dumbbells in your hands. Standing up with shoulders down and back, dumbbells in your hands, and elbows slightly agent, bring your hands and elbows up to shoulder height. Stop the motion when arms are completely parallel to the floor. Slowly lower the weights back down to your side and repeat the move at least twelve times. To make the move more challenging, get in a side plank: balancing with one arm on the ground, body extending and perpendicular to the floor and weight on the side of your feet. Hold a very light dumbbell in your top hand. Your hips should be raised so that your body is in a perfect line. Holding this side plank, slowly raise your upper hand up until the shoulder is at a right angle with the body. Slowly lower that hand back down to the side of your body. Repeat ten to twelve times. Repeat on the other side of the body. This exercise really forces you to use your entire body and both arms for proper form.

Your dietary intake is very important. Don't starve yourself; this will lower your chances of having toned muscles. Eat a small meal every three hours that includes a lean protein, natural carbohydrate such as a fruit or vegetable, and a small amount of fat from nuts or healthy oils. Drink plenty of water. Often times, hunger will disguise true thirst. If you stay hydrated, you will most likely eat less. And try to limit your late night eating to a small, portion-sized snack such as a Jell-O pudding cup, an apple with a few almonds, or a small low-sugar yogurt.

Drink plenty of water to ensure that you are dehydrated. Believe it or not, if you do not drink enough water daily, your body will be more likely to retain water when you finally do drink water.

You should do the recommended amount of cardiovascular exercise, twenty to sixty minutes of exercise most days of the week. Your heart rate should be between 60-85 percent of your maximum heart rate. To determine your age-predicted maximum heart rate, subtract your age from 220. Once you are achieving this recommendation, incorporate resistance training.

Spot reducing does not necessarily work for losing body fat. In other words, doing arm exercises will not necessarily help you lose fat from your arms. However, doing proper exercises can increase your strength and muscle tone and combined with cardiovascular exercise and proper nutrition, you will see the benefits in your arms. Losing body fat in your arms will require a loss of total body fat since none of us can decide where our bodies will lose body fat.

LOSING ALL-OVER BODY FAT

If you are hoping to lose total body fat, then incorporate other exercises such as lunges and squats since they burn many calories and could help you achieve weight and body fat loss. Increasing intensity of all exercises can really improve results as well so be sure to increase the weights and the speed or intensity of your cardio work.

There are countless ways you can lose weight: diet programs, health club memberships, personal training, high-intensity training, and yoga. So how can you know which workout fits you the best and will give you the results you want? It is so difficult to discern all of the information out there: should you focus on diet, exercise, or a combination of both? Is it better to do high intensity exercise or lower intensity exercise? Well, there is a lot of information out there and the best way to find out what is best for you is to compare and contrast the various options you have. Figure out what you can imagine yourself doing long-term, what is enjoyable, and what is realistic for your life.

The key really is that you can lose weight and get healthy in many different ways. Every person adapts and responds differently to different stimuli. One person could get great results from a running plan while another could lose weight performing high intensity weight lifting exercises. The difference can be in motivation and desire to perform that particular type of exercise. As well, our bodies all respond differently so it is good to try a variety of programs and go with what you enjoy, what gives you results, and what you can imagine sustaining over a long period of time.

BODY FAT PERCENTAGE

It is not uncommon for people to lose significant body weight and find out that their body fat percentage is still high. There are many things that could contribute to this. First of all, losing considerable body weight often requires restriction of calorie intake. When calories are drastically restricted, the body reacts by losing weight and the weight lost is both from lean mass and fat mass. If you restrict your calories too low (below 1200 calories a day), then you will most likely cause unwanted muscle mass loss which will affect your total body composition. The weight lost could be from a higher percentage of muscle then from fat. This does not help if your beginning body fat percentage was already higher than it should be. If your lean mass decreases, then your fat mass percentage increases, therefore showing a higher body fat percentage.

You can prevent drastic lean muscle mass loss with resistance training and by not restricting your calorie intake too drastically for an extended period of time. An extended time period of caloric restriction can cause your body's metabolism to slow down. Your brain and organs that secrete appetite hormones are affected by this shift in caloric intake. With a drastic decrease in calories, your body thinks that you are going hungry and will conserve fat tissue for survival.

Why should you care what your body fat percentage is? Risk of heart disease was historically only linked to body weight, total cholesterol, triglycerides, blood pressure, and diabetes. Now, researchers have found that increased body fat percentage, even of normal weight individuals, is linked to higher heart disease risk. According to the American College of Sports Medicine, a forty-year-old man should have a body fat percentage of 21-24 percent to be considered average, and a forty-year-old woman 26-30 percent. The American Council on Exercise states that a woman should be below 31 percent to not be obese and at risk; a man needs to be below 25 percent body fat.

Watch your caloric restriction to ensure appropriate and safe weight loss. It is often recommended to keep calorie restriction to 1500 calories or more a day. If you are trying to lose more weight and want to conserve lean mass, then you should increase your exercise time and intensity. Try to incorporate interval training as this has been shown to decrease belly fat deposition, which is also linked to heart disease risk. Get your dietary fats from healthy sources like nuts, seeds, and oils such as olive and canola. Increase your dietary fiber, vegetable, and fruit intake to fill you up and prevent the feeling of deprivation.

If your goals are improved health and wellness then the result will often be a loss in weight and body fat percentage. Aim to improve your fitness level by training for a 5K, walking daily with a friend, or hiring a trainer to teach you weight training form. Enjoy the feeling of being physically able to complete a workout with ease rather than concentrating solely on the number on the scale.

CALCULATING CALORIE NEEDS

To lose body fat, you need to combine exercise with a diet that is accurate in calories and rich in vegetables and lean protein. Calculate how many calories you need daily to maintain your body weight and aim to spread those calories out with three meals and two to three small snacks a day.

For women, use the formula: BMR = 655 + (4.35 x weight in pounds) + (4.7 x height in inches) - (4.7 x age in years).

For men, use the formula: BMR = 66 + (6.23 x weight in pound) + (12.7 x height in inches) - (6.8 x age in year).

Once you know your BMR (Basal Metabolic Rate), consider your activity level by multiplying it by the appropriate number as follows:

1. If you are sedentary (little or no exercise): Calorie calculation = BMR x 1.2
2. If you are lightly active (light exercise/sports one to three days/week): Calorie calculation = BMR x 1.375
3. If you are moderately active (moderate exercise/sports three to five days/week): Calorie calculation = BMR x 1.55
4. If you are very active (hard exercise/sports six to seven days a week): Calorie calculation = BMR x 1.725
5. If you are extra active (very hard exercise/sports and physical job or exercise 2x a day): Calorie calculation = BMR x 1.9

NON-MODIFIABLE FACTORS IN WEIGHT LOSS

There are many factors that cause or prevent weight gain and weight loss. Physical activity and nutrition are the most common factors but others such as hormone levels and hereditary are also contributors. The most common and also manageable factors are your levels of physical activity and nutritional intake. You can easily control the amount you move each day and the calories that you ingest. However, the way in which your body loses weight and keeps it off is a careful balance of other factors such as hormones and even sleep.

The modifiable factors such as physical activity and lower caloric intake can often lead to weight loss but do not always lead to long-lasting weight loss. Non-modifiable factors such as hormone levels, stress, and sleep are other contributors to difficulty in losing weight and keeping it off. In July 2013, the Journal: Metabolism Clinical and Experimental, Ana Crujeiras, of Complejo Hospitalario Universitario de Santiago in Spain, points to important hormonal factors in weight loss. Appetite hormones such as leptin, ghrelin, and insulin are important in regulating hunger and weight loss. People who tend to gain their weight loss pounds back have higher levels of the hormone ghrelin which acts on the hunger center of the brain, the hypothalamus. The hormone leptin acts on the hypothalamus to inhibit appetite. These hormone levels vary from person to person. Leptin is produced by white adipose fat tissue, brown adipose tissue, some skeletal muscle, mammary glands, and other organs. Leptin is produced and circulates in quantities proportional to fat. Research about the role of leptin in weight loss and appetite control are inconclusive, but there could be a connection between leptin and ghrelin levels and weight loss.

Researchers have also seen some connection between these hormone levels and sleep. Michael Breus, PhD, from the Atlanta School of Sleep Medicine, found that when you do not get enough sleep, it drives levels of leptin down and levels of ghrelin to rise, causing you to not feel as full and satiated after eating. Other studies have shown that men who got more sleep actually weighed more, possibly due to a laziness factor. Men who laid around more, burned fewer calories and therefore had higher weights. This research is inconclusive. So get your shut-eye if you want to keep unnecessary pounds off your waistline. When you do not get enough sleep, you often crave more food that is higher in calories and fat so it will affect weight gain and weight loss.

What are you to do? You can only do what you have control over. Make sure you eat a healthy balanced meal that comes from natural sources every few hours. If getting to bed early is difficult for you, shift your bedtime to fifteen minutes earlier each night. It is best for you to focus on both diet and exercise to lose weight. If you only lower your caloric intake without exercise, you have an increased risk for gaining the weight back. Your daily life should include activity but also try to incorporate resistance training twice a week. The more lean muscle mass you have, the higher metabolism you will have and the less likely you will gain weight when you splurge on a treat every now and then.

Try to not let your weight creep up without getting it under control. Some studies show it is more difficult for people to lose weight if they have gone up and down in weight numerous times. It might be easier to maintain a weight if you stay at the same weight year after year. Going on drastic diets and then reverting back to bad habits can often lead to yo-yo dieting and also yo-yo weight, so be consistent.

CHAPTER 6

NUTRITION

COMFORT FOOD AND NUTRITION

For many people, feeling depressed tends to make them crave comfort food. But feeling blue does not have to cause you to gain weight.

If you are noticing a slow increase in weight, you should look at a few factors. First, has your stress caused you to mindlessly munch? You may find yourself satisfying an emotional need—such as security—for the feelings that food gives you. Do you find yourself returning to the pantry over and over again in the evening just to fill an emotional void? This type of eating is more common when your stress level is high because you are looking for comfort and food can often provide it.

Many of us grew up to associate high fat, creamy, or salty foods with a happy feeling. Can you think back to times when you were growing up and a loved one would comfort you with warm baked cookies or pie? I know I can. So when we feel hopeless, we often turn to food to make us feel better. When we eat those foods, our memories take us back to that feeling of contentment and happiness. Eating comforting foods can also release dopamine, the feel good hormone, in your brain. This creates an actual chemical reaction that causes you to enjoy the food even more and continue the vicious cycle. The problem is that in our current situation, the food only helps for a short time and the depression or difficult situation remains. Therefore, dealing with your emotions with food will not solve problems.

Another thing to look for is a lack of sleep. When we are stressed, especially over long-term problems, we lose sleep over it. When we lose sleep, we misinterpret fatigue with hunger. During the day when you are dragging from missed shut-eye, you probably want to grab some tasty food. Yet you really need more sleep and not more food. This is common for many of us who try to do too much in too few hours a day. We cut out sleep and end up damaging our waistline. So next time you reach for the vending machine, ask yourself, "Am I tired or physically hungry or just trying to fill a void?"

Lastly, if you are dealing with financial issues, you may be buying cheaper foods that are lower in nutritional value. Unfortunately, processed, and oftentimes unhealthy foods are inexpensive. Although it seems like buying easy food will save a few dollars, people often spend just as much money on processed foods for their convenience and forgo healthy options to save time. Instead, spend time cooking with your family in the kitchen; it will save you money and will help foster closeness and will model good behavior to your kids.

I encourage you to look at the long term. If your pocketbook is tighter, try to cut out the unhealthy habits in your life before you cut out buying healthy produce. If you smoke, now would be a good time to quit the habit to save you a lot of money. If you drink a lot of alcohol, you could cut back and save money and calories. If your morning latte is still a daily occurrence, see if you can cut it out or switch to black coffee. That will save you several dollars a day, which translates to over $100 in a month! That could buy you a gym membership and a lot of healthy produce.

VARIETY IN DIET

Eating a variety of foods can help you obtain a healthy lifestyle for many reasons. Eating a variety of foods will help ensure that you are eating all of the vitamins and minerals you need to sustain basic bodily functions and feel good. If you limit your nutritional intake and cut certain food groups out, you risk missing entire vitamins and minerals that are essential to life.

It is fairly common for people in the United States to be stricken with deficiency diseases such as rickets (from lack of vitamin D and possibly lack of calcium) that causes softening of the bones in children, beriberi (from lack of thiamine, B1) a nervous system ailment that causes loss of energy molecules, and scurvy (from lack of Vitamin C). Other disorders can be caused from developmental deficiencies such as spina bifida when a pregnant mother does not have enough folate.

contradicting

These are all deficiency disorders that do not occur very often in America due to our fortified foods and vitamins. Many vitamin and mineral deficiencies have been eradicated in America due to our food system being fortified with essential vitamins. However, eating a variety of minerals, vitamins, and nutrients can help you feel good and function adequately. For example, achieving adequate B vitamins can help you feel energized; they are often found in meat and egg products. Another common mistake people make is not getting enough fat in their diet, which can help support their immune system and improve mood. Anther modern day deficiency is iron deficiency, which can cause anemia (a loss of red blood cells) and fatigue.

Variety can benefit your diet by providing the nutrients you need to feel good. Eating a variety of fruits and vegetables can also provide phytochemicals, which help fight free radicals which damage healthy cells. Colorful vegetables provide a wide variety of phytochemicals that provide immune system protection.

Eating a variety of foods is healthy only when those foods are healthy. Current research points to the problem that eating a wide variety of foods can prevent long term weight loss. Think of the times you walk down the cereal or chip aisle at the grocery store. We have endless options! What does this create when our pantries are stocked full of options? We tend to continue trying different foods until our taste buds feel satisfied and our taste buds usually keep asking for more and different flavors. You may first grab the salty pretzels to satisfy your salt craving, then the sugary cereal to get sweet, and lastly, reach for cheese for that smooth, fatty texture. Variety can sometimes hurt us.

In a study published by the American Society of Clinical Nutrition, it was found that those who ate a more strict variety of foods as well as stuck to their program seven days a week were more successful at losing weight and keeping it off. So even varying your food choices on the weekends can hinder long-term weight loss. Of their 4,000 participants, 20 percent maintained a 10 percent weight loss for two to five years due to healthy eating and exercise habits through the weekend and on holidays. This is in contrast to letting yourself "off the hook" and forgoing exercise and healthy eating on weekends and holidays.

You might find the greatest long-term nutrition success by creating with a professional an eating plan that offers a variety of healthy foods but remains fairly consistent seven days a week. Your diet should be roughly 50-65 percent carbohydrates, 10-15 percent protein, and 10-30 percent fat (healthy fats) as well as eating five to seven fruits and vegetables a day. This will provide a healthy variety of foods. But try to keep your pantry full of healthy options and not ten different types of cereal.

HEALTHY INDULGING

What we eat while enjoying the entertainment of sporting events, movies, or a night out with friends adds to the experience but does usually hamper our nutritional goals.

What can you do to improve your nutritional intake while enjoying tailgating or family movie night—not to mention Christmas dinner? One of the biggest mistakes is eating all prepared foods. If you can manage the time, then home-make anything you can. Making your food helps by allowing you to know what is in your food so you can improve the nutritional content.

For example, instead of buying prepackaged beef patties, make your own out of lean ground sirloin. You can add all the spices and extra touches to make them taste even better. When it comes to buying the fixings, grab whole-wheat buns and natural cheese (not the processed stuff). You can always purchase chips that do not have trans fat and make healthy dips. If you want creamy dips, make them yourself with a package of ranch dip mix and low fat or non-fat sour cream. Other great low fat options are nonfat refried beans and salsa. These are all tasty and are even better options if they will be sitting out; as they will not spoil like mayonnaise-based dips.

If your special event begins early in the morning and you want donuts and pastries, then you can either make them yourself or purchase healthier options. Homemade baked goods tend to taste better and can be made so much healthier, without the trans fat and extra sugar. If you do not have the time or desire to bake, then head to your local bakery. Local bakeries are always open early on Saturdays and you can place your order ahead of time. This allows you to get the freshest foods early if you are on your way out of town.

One of the biggest calorie laden goods for any party, movie theater, or tailgate is the drinks. One common social beverage is beer. Here are some comparisons for you, all for a twelve-ounce serving. A regular Budweiser has 143 calories, a Deschutes Broken Top has 233 calories, a Guinness Draught has 125 calories, and a Coors Light has 102 calories.

You might think that some of these options are not bad for calories but let's imagine you had six over the course of the entire day. If you choose a beer with 150 calories in each bottle/can then you would consume 900 calories. So with nothing else in consideration, including the extra calories in food, you could gain over a pound a month drinking this much one day a week.

On a day when you know you will be eating unhealthy food, eat a healthy breakfast full of fiber and lean protein. This will prevent you from overeating later in the day. Spread out your calories during the whole day. Do not treat the special event like a binge buffet; just eat normal quantities.

If you are at home for a social event, then you really have all the control. Just stock your fridge with healthy options so that you can grab better foods. Try to limit which things you will eat throughout the course of the day so you do not mindlessly eat away at your pantry.

Do not forget exercise! If you know you are eating more calories, then do not skip your workout!

There's no other time like the holiday season for parties and social events. Throughout the holiday season, we are tempted with special treats and dishes that only come around once a year. So we indulge and usually give ourselves a little more leeway with our caloric intake so we can enjoy all of our holiday gatherings without missing out on the great food. But do we really know how many calories we are actually eating and how much exercise it will take to burn off that very special treat? Oftentimes it can be worth enjoying a traditional family treat once a year if it means just a few more minutes at the gym. However, we often underestimate the caloric damage we are doing.

Let's take a closer look at some of our favorite holiday food items and equate that to minutes of exercise needed to break even. (All calories-burned are based on a 145-pound person.)

Food: Pecan pie (no whipping cream)
Nutrition: 530 calories. Fat: 29g
Exercise Equivalent: A tasty slice of pecan pie can increase your need for a good workout! It would take you fifty extra minutes on the elliptical machine to break even with this treat. If you add ½ cup whipped cream to your pie, you will add 200 calories and will need to bump up your cardio session on the elliptical machine to a total of sixty-five minutes!

Food: 1 cup mashed potatoes with gravy
Nutrition: 420 calories. Fat: 22g
Exercise Equivalent: To burn off an extra helping of mashed potatoes and gravy, you would need to rake leaves for at least

two hours. If you want to trim that down to just an hour of leaf raking, cut out the gravy!

Food: 12 oz. of eggnog
Nutrition: 515 calories. Fat: 29g
Exercise Equivalent: It would take you one and a half hours of swimming laps to burn off the one glass of eggnog. If you increase your pace from a moderate intensity to a vigorous one, you could be done burning off the eggnog in forty-five minutes!

Food: Breakfast Casserole
Nutrition: 760 calories. Fat: 46g
Exercise Equivalent: You could ride a bicycle for sixty minutes to burn off the casserole. Unfortunately, the high fat content in the casserole will likely cause lethargy and a tired feeling; making it more difficult to get on the bike! Try to take a smaller portion and add some fresh fruit to your morning holiday breakfast. Limit how much you keep of leftovers so you do not continue eating the same unhealthy breakfast for three days in a row!

Food: Berry pie with ice cream

Nutrition: 740 calories. Fat: 40g

Exercise Equivalent: To burn off one piece of pie and ice cream you would need to do three hours and twenty minutes of light weight training. Weight training is great for developing muscle strength and endurance but make sure you add some cardiovascular exercise to your workout routine too.

If you still want to indulge in the great foods of the holiday season, try to limit your portion sizes and fit in time to exercise regardless of your hectic schedule of shopping, wrapping gifts, and going to holiday festivities. You will be glad you were more aware of the damage that can be done during such a great time of year. By paying closer attention now, you will have less damage control to do later!

STAYING HYDRATED

Hydration is essential for all of us. But if you are exercising and being more active outdoors during the warmer months, you and your family should be well informed about how to stay hydrated and the possible conditions related to dehydration.

If you are not accustomed to the heat, then when the temperature goes up your body may not be well equipped to deal with the excess heat load. Children are at a much higher risk for dehydration due to their less efficient sweating system, which helps most of us cool off. In fact, evaporation of sweat is how your body will get rid of 70-80 percent of your total heat load when under extreme heat situations. So don't be afraid to sweat; it's a necessary part of cooling off.

If the weather is humid, the risk of dehydration and the effects will be much more severe and more fluids will be needed. In a humid environment, the sweat does not easily evaporate into the atmosphere due to the high density of water already in the air. So make sure you wear loose fitting, breathable clothing and hydrate more in hot and humid conditions. If you prepare your body and follow some simple tips, you can improve how you feel and perform in the heat.

It often takes a person at least two weeks to acclimate to exercising in the heat. Exercising first thing in the morning can often give you the coolest temperatures. While acclimating to warmer weather, make sure you have more than enough liquids prior to exercise and during your activity. It is always better to have too much than not enough. Once your body becomes accustomed to the warmer weather, natural physiological responses include: sweating sooner, sweating more, and feeling less fatigued at the same exertion. However, being acclimated to heat does not mean that you can get away with less fluid. You need to make sure you are still replenishing all of your water lost through fluid replacement.

Signs and Symptoms of Common Heat Related Illnesses

HEAT CRAMPS

Signs & Symptoms	Treatment			
Muscular cramping, usually from a lot of sweating	Stop all activity, and sit quietly in a cool place.	Drink clear juice or a sports beverage.	Do not return to demanding activity for a few hours after the cramps subside. Further activity could lead to heat exhaustion or heat stroke.	Seek medical attention for heat cramps if they do not stop after one hour.

HEAT EXHAUSTION

Signs & Symptoms	Treatment
Heavy sweating , Paleness Muscle cramps , Tiredness Weakness, Dizziness Headache, Nausea or vomiting Fainting	Seek medical attention immediately if the symptoms are severe or the victim has heart problems or high blood pressure. Otherwise, cool off the victim, and seek medical attention if the symptoms worsen or last longer than one hour.

HEAT STROKE

Signs & Symptoms

Treatment

Have someone call for immediate medical assistance and begin cooling the victim:

An extremely high body temperature (above 103°F, orally)

Red, hot, and dry skin (no sweating)

Rapid, strong pulse

Throbbing headache

Dizziness

Nausea

Confusion

Unconsciousness

Get the victim to a shady area.

Cool the victim quickly using whatever you can – put them in a tub or shower of cool water; spray them with cool water from a garden hose; sponge them with cool water.

Monitor body temperature, and continue cooling efforts until the body temperature drops to 101-102°F.

If there is vomiting, make sure the airway remains open by turning the victim on his or her side.

General Hydration Recommendations

The Institute of Medicine determined that an adequate intake (AI) for men is roughly 3 liters (about thirteen cups) of total beverages a day. The AI for women is 2.2 liters (about nine cups) of total beverages a day.

Recommendations for Fluid Before, During, and After Exercise

- **Before:** consume approximately seventeen to twenty fluid ounces of water or a sports drink two to three hours before exercise and seven to ten fluid ounces of water or a sports drink ten to twenty minutes before exercise.

- **During:** How much to drink during your exercise bout is highly dependent on how much water you are losing. The best way to measure that is to weigh yourself immediately before exercise and then immediately after. For every pound you have lost, you should consume sixteen to twenty ounces of water. If you drank liquids during this trial period, then add that liquid to the sixteen ounces per pound to ensure proper fluids. The NATA (National Athletic Trainers Association) recommends seven to ten fluid ounces every ten to twenty minutes. This can be difficult to carry on you, so you might want to plan a route or activity near a fresh water source.

- **After:** Compensate for urine losses incurred during the rehydration process and drink about 25 to 50 percent more than sweat losses to assure optimal hydration four to six hours after the event.

If you are exercising for more than an hour in extreme heat or humidity, then you should include electrolytes and carbohydrates into your beverage. Most sports drinks have the appropriate 6 percent carbohydrate drink with 0.3 to 0.7 g/L of sodium. If you are losing electrolytes in your sweat, it is imperative that you include them in your rehydration solutions so you do not dilute your blood plasma, which leads to a condition called hyponatremia.

Preventing Heat Related Illness

- Drink more fluids, regardless of your activity level. Don't wait until you're thirsty to drink.
- Don't drink liquids that contain alcohol or large amounts of sugar; these actually cause you to lose more body fluid.
- Wear lightweight, light-colored, loose-fitting clothing
- Limit your outdoor activity to morning and evening hours
- Try to rest often in shady areas
- Protect yourself from the sun by wearing a wide-brimmed hat (this also keeps you cooler).

CHAPTER 7

PREVENTING AND MANAGING INJURIES

Stretching and flexibility exercises have long been prescribed for decreasing injuries and for improving flexibility. There are many different types of stretching. There are ballistic, static, and dynamic stretching. Ballistic stretching is when you bounce through a stretch. An example would be leaning down to stretch your hamstrings and letting your back go up and down. Static stretching is when you hold a particular stretch for a time period. An example of static stretching would be leaning down to stretch your hamstrings, reaching a stopping point and holding it for fifteen to thirty seconds. Lastly, dynamic stretching is when you move through a large range of motion that mimics various activities that you might participate in during your workout. An example of dynamic stretching would be slow, partial lunges or skipping before a run.

Most of the research out there advises against ballistic (bouncing) stretching at any time since it can increase your risk of injury by pulling a muscle past its point of flexibility. Research for static stretching benefits goes back decades and is still a large part of many athletic and training programs. Static stretching can increase the muscle fiber length if performed properly and after the muscle is adequately warmed-up.

A muscle fiber is an elastic and plastic region. In the beginning of a stretch or increased range of motion, the muscle will come back to its original length when you relax. If you go beyond the elastic range, you start deformation of tissue and enter the plastic region where you can, hopefully, increase the muscle's length. After a muscle is sufficiently warm—after a workout—is the best time to statically stretch the muscle to try to increase the muscle length. Hold a stretch for a minimum of fifteen seconds and as much as sixty seconds in a range that is slightly uncomfortable, not painful, and at a range that allows you to continue normal breathing. If you statically stretch a cold muscle, you could possibly injure the muscle tissue and you performance might also suffer. Static stretching tends to slow reaction of proprioceptors in your muscles called muscle spindles and Golgi tendon organs that prevent you from over stretching a muscle and damaging it. If you statically stretch for a long period of time then you will begin to trick these proprioceptors into slowing their reactivity and therefore could cause for a decrease in neuromuscular (nerve) recruitment and firing. Therefore, static stretching should be left to being performed after a workout when muscles are warm and you are done with any athletic performance.

Prior to working out, dynamic stretching is the best way for you to improve your flexibility and performance as well as reduce the chance of injury. Once you have jogged or walked for roughly five minutes or more, you can begin a dynamic stretching routine. Some good dynamic stretches are slow, controlled lunges with a high knee in between: pace ten lunges forward with a high knee and back, alternating legs. Another good dynamic stretch is skipping, or lateral karaoke. By performing controlled movements that mimic large joint ranges of motions, you can increase range of motion during your workout, warm up your muscles, and decrease injury. So depending on what your sport is, consider different dynamic stretches that mimic sport movement.

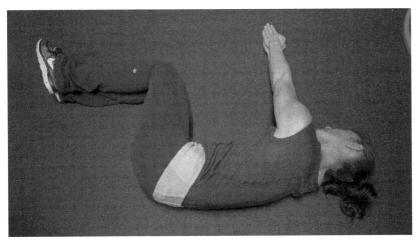

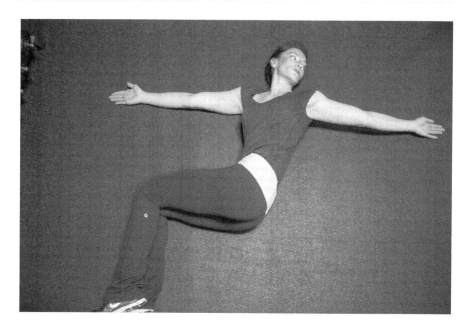

If nothing else, remember that some people are more flexible than others based on genetics and joint specific issues such as arthritis, inflammation, and muscle and fat mass in that area. You can train for increased flexibility, but you can also be too mobile (hypermobile). If you overstretch continuously, and your joints are extremely flexible, you could be sacrificing stability and could increase a risk for injury or subluxation of joints.

Stretch within your limits, after warming up, and with deep, normal breathing.

RECOVERING QUICKLY FROM INJURIES

As people age they tend to get injured more, with common injuries to the back, neck, and shoulders. It can take a long time to heal and get back to a regular physical activity pattern.

The best option is to prevent the injury from occurring in the first place. Prevention involves many factors, including regular resistance, core, and balance training. Most back injuries could be prevented from developing a stronger core (abdominal wall, back muscular, hips, and gluteus muscles) and better mechanics while lifting in the gym or everyday items. If your core work involves just floor crunches, then you are not working the entire core that will support your low back. Instead, get on a stability ball to do crunches, do planks to strengthen stabilization muscles, or try Pilates moves that will strengthen your transverse abdominus. Your transverse abdominus is the most inner abdominal muscle that acts as a corset; you can feel it tighten when you pull in your navel. Next, make sure that when you perform resistance training moves or even when you lift a heavy grocery bag, that you always keep your core tight and back neutral. Regular exercise and proper mechanics can really help in preventing injuries.

What do you do once an injury has already occurred? You must be proactive in the healing process. No matter what the injury you should keep a close eye on it. A few days of rest could help alleviate some immediate pain; also try to ice the injured area for fifteen to twenty minutes at a time to reduce swelling. If the strain or pain does not subside within a few days, see a physician or physical therapist to rule out any major injuries.

Many people make mistakes once they get injured. They often immobilize the injured area for too long. What occurs, most often with the neck and back, is that sustained immobilization causes reduced range of motion and reduced strength. When you go back to a normal exercise routine, you now have less range of motion and strength, which sets you up for another injury. Aim to gently move the injured area through a safe, pain-free range of motion multiple times a day to encourage blood flow that will help the injury heal while diminishing the chances of losing strength.

Once you have a large pain-free range of motion, you need to slowly rehabilitate it back to normal function. Do not rush this portion and start lifting heavy weights or jumping into a competitive game of basketball! Keep your motions controlled and slow. This is also true for prevention. Rapid movement while lifting weights or objects can increase your risk of muscle strain and injury so keep your moves slow.

If a particular area is injured for a lengthy period of time, do not let this keep you on the couch for too long. This will cause a quick decrease in cardiovascular function and muscular strength. Recurring injuries will keep your sedentary and cause you to be more susceptible to injury as well as a less conditioned person. So find an alternative form of exercise that allows you to still work the rest of your body and stay in shape. If you hurt your back, try the pool; if you have a knee injury, you can still do an arm bike and arm resistance training. Do not let an injury of one part of your body cause you to let the rest of your body go. If you are not sure what exercises are safe for your particular injury and the progression of healing, consult a physical therapist to help guide you. You are most often better off moving then not moving, so try to work with your body to heal. Just hoping and waiting for a recovery is not always the best bet.

INTENSE WORKOUTS WITHOUT PAIN

Higher intensity workouts result in a higher caloric burn and therefore, a greater caloric deficit, which leads to weight loss. So if you are walking now, increasing intensity is often toward running. Other people try kickboxing, aerobics classes, and even plyometrics that involve a lot of jumping. For people with joint pain, intense workouts often feel unrealistic. Many high-intensity exercises that involve jumping and impact can cause joint pain in your knees and other susceptible areas like your low back.

When you think of lower intensity exercises you imagine walking, recumbent bicycle, water aerobics, and yoga. All of these exercises can be done in a more intense but pain-free way for your joints.

Walking workouts can increase in intensity by increasing the incline on the treadmill or find a walking route that has many hills. This will increase your caloric burn by quite a bit without much added jarring. As well, yoga can be very difficult in intensity and burn calories if you are performing a more intense type of yoga such as Ashtanga yoga. If you like cycling, try a spinning class, as this does not often increase joint loading (if the bike is adjusted properly), but will increase total caloric burn.

Now, here is where many more avid gym goers get stuck. If you are a runner, you cannot simply continue adding up running miles without possibly causing increased joint loading. And plyometric drills can often help with weight loss and toning but jumping workouts put increased stress on your knee joints. So what other things could you do to improve your chances of losing weight and getting in an intense workout?

There has been increasing research on deep water running and the caloric expenditure of that activity compared to on-land running. A company by the name of AQX has researched and found that if you wear an aqua shoe and lean slightly forward while running in deep water, you will burn as much, if not more, calories than running on land. And you will have much less impact and reaction forces than you do on land. You can use an aqua flotation belt to keep you afloat but a buoyancy suit might help provide better running form. An aqua belt can cause you to lean back, which is not like the form on land. An aqua jogging suit, which you can buy from AQX, allows your body's center of mass to be distributed properly while you are under water to provide kinematics (form) while water running. This is a great alternative to increasing running intensities and miles on land, which can exacerbate joint pain. You can also do jumping movements and lateral movements in the water with the same results.

Although high intensity exercise does increase total caloric burn for that specific workout, remember that weight loss is a mathematical calorie in and calorie out equation. You have to burn more calories than you put in your body. Eat a healthy, clean diet and try to burn at least 1500 calories a week. That is the minimum recommended number of calories you should burn to improve health according the American College of Sports Medicine. For weight loss, you should increase your caloric burn up to 2,000 to 3,000 calories burned a week. Be careful with a high-impact, high-intensity workout if you are feeling pain in your joints. Some people's joints are more prone to a painful inflammation response. Do what you can do and modify your program based on your personal goals and abilities.

RUNNER'S KNEE

Chondromalacia, also termed "runner's knee," is a condition in which you can feel pain within and around the kneecap. The pain stems from irritation of the underside of the kneecap, called the patella. The smooth cartilage that lines the underside of the patella can become irritated by the patella not tracking appropriately and rubbing on one side or the other of the bone lying beneath it. Damage to the deep layer of the cartilage can cause pain during bending movements and after exercise. Unlike arthritis in which the cartilage undergoes degeneration from disease and is mostly irreversible, cartilage irritation from chondromalacia can repair.

Although men can feel patello-femoral pain from chondromalacia, it is more common in women. This is due to anatomical differences; women's hip and knee joints align at a more severe angle, causing a higher likelihood that the patella tracks improperly and cause irritation of the cartilage. Men can incur the same condition if they have muscle imbalances that perpetuate the problem. Oftentimes people create tight inner thigh muscles (also called adductors) and weak outer thigh muscles (called abductors) and this creates abnormal tracking and movement at the knee during movement.

The first line of defense would be to stop the irritation. Most often, that means resting and taking time away from high impact activities such as running and jumping movements. This will allow the inflammation to go down which should also decrease the pain. You could also ice for fifteen minutes at a time after any exercise. You should be able to initially do pool exercise whether it is swimming laps or pool walking. The pool is a great option for low-impact activity that will keep you moving but without impact on your knee. The next step would be some rehabilitative therapy. I highly suggest you contact a reputable physical therapist. Private clinic physical therapists can assist you without referrals and can best diagnose and treat a condition such as chondromalacia. Strengthening and stretching of the hamstrings and quadriceps can be beneficial in treating your symptoms and prevent reoccurrence. With permission from your physician, non-steroidal anti-inflammatory drugs can help decrease pain and inflammation.

Make sure that you continue moving your body in some fashion. Movement of joints actually increases joint lubrication, bringing healthy fluids in for healing and moving waste and toxins out. So movement is good, just make sure your therapist approves your exercise program. It is often recommended that you stay away from deep knee bends, quadriceps leg extensions that cause high torque on the knee, and high impact moves. Instead, opt for multi-joint movements such as body weight squats and walking.

Surgery is not normally the best scenario for this type of condition. Adequate physical therapy and proper exercise can improve function and limit symptoms often better than surgical intervention.

Chondromalacia is not a normal condition so do not ignore the signs of joint tenderness and pain. If the pain persists, make sure you are giving yourself adequate time to recover and rest and make sure that you do not progress too quickly. For example, if you have been running an average of two miles a day, do not jump up your Saturday run to ten miles. Allow your body and muscles to adapt to the intensity that you are asking it to perform. You have to invest in the treatment if you want to decrease pain. Make sure you are an active participant in the treatment plan to stop the pain and prevent it from happening again.

KNEE PAIN

Knee injuries are difficult to self-diagnose so I urge you to get a physician or physical therapist to test and diagnose any potential knee injury. Injury to the knee could be from a variety of musculoskeletal variables.

The knee has many muscles, tendons, and ligaments that provide strength and stability to the joint. When the knee is stressed through joint loading, twisting, or cutting movements, many components can be injured. Within the knee joint you have menisci (two within each knee joint), which can be damaged with pounding and twisting movements. The menisci are not well supplied with blood which can increase time to heal and often requires surgical repair if the injury is severe enough. Twisting while loading the knee can injure the interior cruciate ligaments. Twisting the knee joint and cutting can injure the anterior cruciate ligament (ACL). If you strain your knee with the lower limb (tibia) moving too far backward, you can injure the posterior cruciate ligament (PCL). The ACL is the most commonly injured knee ligament and often causes intense rehabilitation or surgery to repair the strength and integrity of the joint. If you feel that your knee is unstable during squatting and single leg stepping movements, you might have injured your ACL and should get an exam.

Quadriceps and patellar tendon soreness could be an overuse injury and might simply require rest time, icing, and improving muscular imbalance. Many athletes and physically active people tend to have imbalances between the medial and lateral quadriceps as well as hamstring imbalances. Overtime this can cause your patellar tendon to track improperly, creating knee swelling and pain. Ice for twenty minutes each time you ice. Make sure you warm up adequately before physical activity.

Braces can help support your knee but the problem with going to the store and buying your own brace is that you are essentially selecting a brace without knowing which one will help your particular problem. Certain braces could actually increase the muscular imbalances, which could increase your pain and cause further injury. So getting a physician or therapist recommendation for a brace is recommended. Taking non-steroidal inflammatory drugs (NSAIDS) can also help reduce inflammation and decrease pain and swelling, however you should get permission from your physician to take such over-the-counter medicines if you are on other medicines or are taking NSAIDS on a recurring basis.

If your knee pain continues with rest and icing, you might need to get an exam. Normal muscle soreness should not last more than a week. If pain persists, get it checked out and stop performing activities that increases pain until you get treatment.

GOLFER'S SHOULDER

Most golfers encounter an injury a two per season and they can vary from low back pain to knee injury. A common injury is "golfer's shoulder," due to the excessive range of motion you require from your shoulder during each swing.

Most golfers lack a wide range of motion in their shoulder, especially in external rotation (when your arm is traveling away from the center of the body). External rotation occurs during both your back swing and your follow through and allows for a very vulnerable positioning of your shoulder. This shoulder joint that is externally rotated is called your glenohumeral joint and is the ball and socket joint of your shoulder (where your arm bone, the humerus head, sits in the glenoid fossa, or socket joint, of your scapula). This joint is highly moveable but what it has in mobility it lacks in stability. That means this joint is highly open to injury.

Oftentimes when someone has a limited range of motion, they compensate for it with other musculature in the area. Also, you have many ligaments that run through a very small space in your shoulder joint that can get impinged and push on the nerve. That can cause some serious pain if the ligaments keep getting pushed as you might do with continuing to play round after round through the pain. More inflammation causes more pushing on the nerve and more pain. If you feel severe pain when rotating your shoulder, then try taking it easy for a few days without asking your shoulder to work through any pain.

To prevent this type of injury, exercise your rotator cuff muscles and stretch your shoulder out to improve range of motion. The best way to start is by using thin elastic tubing. The most common colors given to the weaker elastic tubing are yellow and green. You can often find them in the gym weight room or at your local exercise equipment store. Try performing external and internal rotation movements while holding on to the handle of one end of the tubing. Have the other end strapped around a sturdy support. Perform fifteen repetitions in both directions. Then perform the following stretches and repeat twice:

For improving the range of motion of your shoulder joint, move in all directions that your shoulder moves on the course.

First, stretch your chest by placing your forearms at a ninety-degree angle against a door jam. Then gently let your body fall through the doorway as you feel the stretch in your chest. Hold for thirty seconds and repeat. Make sure you breathe throughout.

Second, stretch the backside of your shoulder by grabbing a bar or weight machine at shoulder height. If you are trying to stretch the back of your right shoulder then grab the support with your right hand and your right arm crossing in front of your chest. Then slowly pull your body away while still hanging on. You should feel this stretch across your back.

Lastly, you can enlist the help of a partner to help stretch your shoulder in extreme internal and external rotation; make sure they help you gently. Back off if you feel any pain.

As the previous exercises and stretches become easier, then you can progress to the cable machine. Attach a rope attachment to a weight cable machine on the lowest (closest to ground) setting. With a very light weight, try and mimic your normal golf swing in a slow motion. As uncomfortable as it might seem, do this with your non-dominant side as well. This will help ensure that your body is equally strong and that you do not develop tight musculature on one side while weakening the other. Do two sets of twelve repetitions. Instead of increasing the resistance, work on increasing the speed of your swing.

If pain in your shoulder seems to crop up after a round on the course or at the driving range, then try icing the area afterward. This will help lessen inflammation and also pain. If pain persists during activities of daily living then you need to see your physician or physical therapist to rule out any major joint injuries that will require more thorough rehabilitation.

HANDLING MUSCLE SORENESS

Some muscle soreness is normal. You should feel sore if your program is new or if you are coming back after a long drought away from exercise. If you are properly changing your routine, you will notice that the first week of a new program will cause you soreness as if you hadn't been working out at all. This is normal and actually good for your body. Soreness only becomes a problem if it lingers past a week or so. Your body should start to again slowly adapt to the new program after a couple of weeks.

It is best to change your program (lifting or cardio) at least every four to six weeks to prevent a plateau, which would cause your body to stop changing physically. Our bodies are very good at adapting to the demands we place on it. If you continue challenging it, you will create physiological change.

If you're feeling sore and wonder if it's okay to workout, ask yourself these questions:

- Is the pain dull or sharp? Sharp pain indicates injury.
- Do only certain movements cause pain in a joint? If yes, you could have an injury.
- Does the pain subside once I have warmed up? If no, then you might have an injury; muscle soreness and tightness will decrease after a good warm-up.
- Am I still functional? In other words, can I still do the movement, even with less strength?

It is important that you recognize the difference between soreness and pain. If you are experiencing continuous sharp pain or only pain with certain joint movements, then you could have an injury that will require you to see a sports medicine doctor.

There are ways to decrease muscle soreness after a workout. One of the most fundamental things you can do is warm up and cool down. Every workout should include some sort of ramping up and ramping down. This can be ten minutes or so of light cardiovascular and stretching moves. It is always a good idea to warm up with full body movements before stretching. Stretching cold muscles could actually cause muscle strain.

Also, make sure that your exercise form is correct. This might not prevent soreness but it will prevent injury. If you are not sure how to use a piece of equipment, ask a certified professional, not the muscle-laden guy who just looks like he knows.

The next steps of preventing soreness are in the recovery phase. Recovery begins the second you stop exercising. Once you are done with your cool down and stretching, your body is in a state of recovery. Many people do not do what their body needs to prevent soreness.

One of the most important aspects of your recovery is food. You have to eat! The most important time to eat is immediately after your workout (fifteen to thirty minutes after the workout). If you are headed back to work or running errands, come to the gym prepared with some sort of post-workout meal.

The best post-workout meal consists of a high-glycemic carbohydrate and easily digestible protein. The high-glycemic carbohydrate will help replenish your glycogen stores, which is where your muscles derive their energy. Therefore, this portion of your post-workout meal is just as important as the protein. Research has shown that your muscles can uptake the most carbohydrates and store them as glycogen immediately after exercise. A good example would be a banana, an apple, or potatoes. A 150-pound person would need 50-150 grams of carbohydrates after exercise. A sport drink works okay if you have nothing else, but real food is always better. A good example of easily digestible protein would be 100% whey protein or lean chicken breast. This post-workout meal will help you recover from your workout and get you ready for the next one.

If you are doing all of the right things and are simply feeling sore from a tough workout, then try to hit the gym. Perform a light cardiovascular exercise such as walking followed by a deep stretching activity to loosen any tight muscles. A few days after the tough workout, you might be able to add more resistance to your workout and not worry about injury.

HANDLING EXERCISE PAIN

Muscular fatigue is a common and actually expected part of exercise. But it can be really hard to know if the pain you are experiencing is harmful or helpful. Our bodies have pain receptors to prevent us from injuring ourselves. These receptors are in overdrive when you put your body beyond where it is comfortable. Different modes of exercises can produce different types of pain and fatigue. For a new exerciser, it's difficult to discern between injury producing pain and helpful limit pushing.

Exercise serves the purpose of improving your health and fitness capabilities. To improve your fitness, you have to provide a stimulus—intensity that pushes your body slightly past what is comfortable. If you only did what was comfortable or normal, then you would likely not see a change.

The term used for increasing the intensity of what your demand of your body is called progressive overload. Progressive overload allows your body to experience slight discomfort and even connective tissue damage. For example, when you lift weights, your muscles might actually be slightly damaged as seen in micro trauma tears in muscle fibers. In your rest time, the muscles recover and rebuild even stronger muscular tissue. That is how strength training increases your muscle size and strength.

You definitely need adequate rest time in between exercise sessions to allow connective tissue to regenerate and repair. If you go hard day after day, then you will be continually damaging tissue and not giving it adequate time to heal. If you are currently working hard back-to-back days then you might need to insert some rest days; any pain you might experience could be overuse injury.

Muscle soreness might peak twenty-four to forty-eight hours after a tough workout. Instead of lying on the couch, treat the soreness with movement. Go for a slow walk to loosen muscles and move fluid into the joints. Strictly resting can stiffen you up more.

Cardiovascular exercise strengthens your heart muscle and improves lung function. If you experience severe chest pain, dizziness, or shortness of breath without increasing intensity, it could be a sign of heart problems. However, slight discomfort during higher intensity exercise could be your pushing of the ventilator and respiratory threshold. Everyone's threshold varies and can be improved with cardiovascular exercise. Some discomfort might be experienced during training when you are going a little faster or at an incline. Severe pain and discomfort could warrant you seeing a cardiologist for a stress test to determine if there are underlying contraindications.

The first questions to ask yourself when you experience exercise related pain are: what type of exercise am I doing, and how intense am I pushing? If you are doing a primarily non-weight bearing activity like swimming, water aerobics, or even the elliptical machine, you should not feel severe joint pain. Harmful joint pain might feel like sharp pain during certain ranges of motion and can often be worse at the beginning of the activity, before there is adequate fluid movement in the joint. Once you are warmed up, joint pain can subside. However, if you are pushing yourself into severe ranges of motion, joints can signal pain to protect you.

Sharp pain during various movements often signals injury within the joint, tendon, or ligament. If you feel weakness at the beginning of a workout you could have muscular injury. However, fatigue toward the end of a set of weight training exercises could be signaling muscular fatigue. Fatigue might feel like weakness towards the end of a workout. If you reach fatigue before reaching a prescribed repetition or set, then lower the weight you are lifting so you do not hurt yourself. Do not keep pushing past fatigue if you do not have a spotter, as you could injure yourself.

If you tend to come and go with exercise, you might experience fatigue and discomfort each time you exercise. If you can stick to a routine of exercising at least three days a week, you could lessen your pain and soreness.

FOOT PAIN

There are many reasons for this foot pain while exercising. If you are experiencing foot pain, the first and most important thing to determine is if your shoes are supportive enough.

First assess if your shoes are the right type of shoes for the anatomy of your foot. If your feet have high arches, then you need shoes that have appropriate arch support, therefore dramatically reducing the risk of your arches falling. High arched feet also need a firm and sturdy lateral/side portion of the shoes so that your foot does not supinate too much. That means you do not want your foot to fall outward to the outside part of your foot too much. If you have flat feet or fallen arches, you also need support in your arches so that your foot does not pronate too much, which occurs when your foot falls toward the inside of your foot. This can cause internal rotation of your calf, which can cause many more problems.

The most common source of pain in the foot during exercise is due to nerves such as the plantar flexor nerve being irritated or pinched during movement. This can occur when your feet are not used to impact aerobic exercise and the muscles inflame, causing pressure on the nerves that travel down your leg and to the foot.

One problem with machines like the stair master and the elliptical machine is that your foot does not get a lot of movement. Your foot stays predominantly on the step the entire time you are exercising. This is great for providing aerobic exercise without too much impact but it does prevent proper blood circulation in your feet. The movement of the foot during walking and running helps blood circulation and venous return, which is returning blood to the heart and lungs for oxygenation. Without proper flexing and extending of the foot during exercise, you tend to lose a lot of this vasoconstriction (vein contraction that pushes blood back to the heart).

The lack of normal movement of the foot when you are on the stair master and elliptical machine can be combined with other problems such as too tight shoelaces. When your shoelaces are too tight, there is pressure on the plantar and foot nerves, which can cause a feeling of numbness and pain. If you are experiencing a feeling of numbness or tingling in your foot during exercise, it could be that you are losing proper blood circulation in your foot. This is obviously the issue if you do not have numbness or tingling when walking on the treadmill or riding a bicycle.

If you experience foot pain each time you exercise on a machine, it doesn't necessarily mean you need to quit doing that particular exercise. Instead try to loosen your shoelaces so blood can circulate more freely to your foot and toes. If this does not seem to help, then you might have to consciously raise your feet every now and then when making strides forward on an exercise machine. This could improve blood circulation and reduce numbness and pain. If the feeling continues, spend a shorter amount of time on this machine and alternate time on the treadmill. For example, do ten minutes on one and switch to the other and go back and forth like this until you have completed the entire duration of the workout.

If you are new to walking longer distances, you could simply be building up skin tissue calluses. That is common if your feet are simply not used to the miles and rubbing in a shoe. Check to see if your feet are creating blisters after you walk longer distances. If you are walking in warmer weather your feet could be more prone to abrasive problems such as heat rash and blisters. I recommend moisture-wicking fabric socks to eliminate sweat building up in your shoes. As well, make sure that your shoes have ample space for your feet to move around during walking. You do not want shoes to be too tight which can cause blisters on your toes and heels. But if your shoes are much too big then you could also get too much movement and this could increase your risk for blisters as well. It is commonly recommended that you wear a walking shoe that is laced snugly but maybe a half size bigger than you would normally wear to give your toe box enough room.

It is also recommended that you wear a proper walking shoe. Running shoes should not be worn for strictly walking as they are designed for different movement, just as walking shoes shouldn't be used for strictly running. Go to a local shoe store to have a trained professional watch you walk and provide you with the best shoe for your stride and foot and arch shape. If blisters continue to be a problem, you could be building up calluses. To prevent blisters, after getting the right socks and shoes, you could add some Vaseline to your feet. Prep your feet by rubbing Vaseline between your toes and any spots that might rub a lot during a longer walk. Then carefully put on your socks and shoes.

If pain persists and you begin to notice pain during your walk, you might want to see a podiatrist or other physician to rule out other problems. Persons with peripheral artery disease (PAD) will often get pain in their lower extremities with exertion. Most often, pain is present in the back of the thigh and down the lower calf, but pain could refer down to your toes. PAD is when arteries in the lower limbs become narrowed or clogged with plaque or fatty deposits. Narrowing of arteries in the lower limbs is often associated with clogging and hardening of the arteries around the heart and can be a sign of current or future heart disease. Often pain associated with PAD is increased with increasing exercise intensity and is relieved with rest and leg elevation. However, exercise has been found to be a great treatment for those with PAD and can actually help relieve symptoms if the intensity is appropriate. If the pain is in the lower limbs and your feet, compression socks could help by increasing the return of blood to your heart and decreasing cramping. If you have pain during exercise, it is always recommended to see your physician.

Before worrying about a serious disease, try getting good socks and shoes. Also, increase your mileage gradually to allow your muscles and even your skin to adjust to the increase in motion.

The most important thing is that you do not let this situation stop you from exercising or enjoying it! Try to find a solution or find another form of exercise that you enjoy just as much.

OSTEOARTHRITIS

Exercise is extremely important for patients with osteoarthritis. It might seem like a joint disease would be worsened by exercise, yet research shows that those who exercise have a lessened severity of the symptoms.

One of the greatest benefits of exercise is lessened body weight. Excess body weight can increase the pain and effects of the disease. More body weight means more pounding on your joints with each and every step. With more activity, you will burn calories and lose weight, and therefore improve your joint pain.

Movement can help improve joint synovial fluid distribution and allow for less stiffness. If you have extremely weak muscles, you may find that the pain is worsened with exercise. This can be due to improper tracking of a joint, particularly the knee. If you feel that you have an unstable joint or weakness during particular movements, see a physical therapist to help correct any muscular imbalances. With re-education of muscles, you can lessen the overuse inflammation that is occurring in your affected joints.

If pain persists after exercise, you might need less jarring activities and possibly some preventive measures taken. Make sure you have a prolonged warm up to improve blood and fluid flow. Also, stretch your entire body. Stretching your body can help alleviate particular muscle tightness that can lead to improper movement and therefore joint pain. If your doctor warrants it, you could try taking a non-steroidal inflammatory drug (NSAID) to decrease inflammation. This could lessen the pain during and following exercise. Research has even shown that exercise can delay or even prevent the need for surgery. Hip and knee function have also been seen to improve with exercise.

One of the best and most often recommended exercises for osteoarthritis patients is a pool workout. If swimming laps is too vigorous, then try simple water walking. While staying in a pool that allows you to touch for the length of the pool, walk as you would outdoors. Take your time and allow your body to use the water as resistance. You can also try a water aerobics class. These classes are designed to provide adequate resistance exercises while minimizing joint jarring and painful movements.

Common complaints about pool workouts are getting in and out of the pool, being uncomfortable in swimwear around other people, or just the hassle of showering at the gym. Remember that you are not alone. Many people have these same fears or did at one time. It takes experience to feel more comfortable. As you develop a routine, your fears will diminish. Also remember that to change your body you have to change your actions. Take a chance and see how great you feel after exercise and it might be worth it.

Also try basic stretching or range of motion exercises. Get a light resistance band to do basic arm and leg movements. Hire a personal trainer or physical therapist to help guide you through the movements the first few times.

Do not overdo it. If your joint pain persists for more than two hours after exercise then you could be over-exercising. Cut back your intensity and duration so that you feel good when you have completed your routine. Remember that some exercise is better than none. Take it slow.

If you decide to try weight training, stick to multi-joint, full body movements. You want to train your body the way you expect it to move during the day. Stay away from knee extensions, knee curls, and arm curls. Try full body standing up, sitting down type movements. Minimize your range of motion if you need and work on your stretching so that you can move with more ease.

Here are some suggestions if you struggle with motivation. Find a buddy who will meet you at the gym and even exercise with you. A spouse or friend is great, but if you can find someone with similar situations then you will feel more at ease. The Arthritis Foundation sponsors an exercise program called PACE (People with Arthritis Can Exercise). You can look up their programs and where they are offered at www.arthritis.org.

I encourage you to write down your efforts and successes. For some people, to see their accomplishment on paper is more motivating than a number on the scale. Reward yourself for exercising at least three times a week.

If you still find that any exercising at all is excruciating, you need the guidance of a licensed and well-experienced physical therapist. Finding guidance and help to find the root cause of your pain is essential if you want to decrease osteoarthritis pain and improve your mobility and health. Do not give up. Be proactive and find a professional who can help you.

POSTURE

Appropriate posture is a learned habit. With time and bad habits, it is easy to fall into a slumped position that puts you at risk for back injury, pain, and other bodily effects such as shortness of breath. How is one to know if they have good posture or not? How do we end up having such bad posture and how can we fix it? Improved posture will improve athletic performance, decrease back pain, improve effectiveness at work, and even improve self-confidence. Physical therapist Jeffrey Blanchard says, "With optimal posture, you are in your balanced and neutral alignment. Muscles and joints don't have to work as hard when you are optimally aligned and you will have greater tolerance to positions with optimal posture, such as sitting at your desk all day."

What causes bad posture?

Many people spend their days slumped forward while driving, typing on the computer, or doing dishes. If you exercise slouched, you make the problem worse. Over time as you slouch forward, gravity tends to increase the pull downward and your posture worsens. It requires conscious effort to maintain the appropriate spinal alignment to prevent any back pain or injury. While slouching forward, the middle and lower back will have vertebrae and discs that are being strained in ways not meant for long-term position. You should naturally have a small curve going inward in your lower back. As you slouch you can tell that your lower back rounds out and this can cause excess pressure on discs and boney vertebrae. As well, as your chin starts to wander out in front of your chest and your shoulders round forward, your upper back muscles become elongated and tight. This will give you stress headaches and likely cause tension. Poor posture could even lead to poor breathing as your slouched shoulders reduce the space your lungs can inflate.

Posture Check:

Stand in front of a blank doorway (the door jams and framing can help you use them as a guide for a straight reference). Wear shorts and a tank top to get a good idea of what your actual body looks like. Have a friend take photos of you standing with views from the front, side, and rear. Make sure to stand relaxed. When looking at the picture you should take note of the following that would signify good posture.

- Your ears, shoulders, hips and ankles should all line up vertically.
- Does your low back arch inward or hunch outward?
- Does your chin jet out in front of your chest?
- Are your knees going inward/outward or hyperextending?

If you said yes to any of these, then you need to correct your posture.

Posture exercises you can do daily:

Chin tucks. This might feel silly to most people but it can make a huge difference in your posture and tension headaches. Sit up tall and pull your chin back (making a double chin). Hold for five seconds and repeat at least ten times at each sitting. You can repeat as many times as you would like.

Chest opening. Lie on your back and drop your right knee over your left leg and twist your spine while opening up your right arm and keeping it flat on the ground. Hold for twenty seconds and repeat on each side.

Bent T's. Either lying flat on your chest on a bench or carefully with a flat back leaning forward, raise your straight arms up and out to the sides as if making a T with your body and arms. Hold at the top for five seconds and slowly lower. Repeat ten times. This will open up your chest and strengthen your shoulders and upper back muscles.

Active hip stretch. Kneel on one knee and have the other leg bent at 90 degrees at the hip and knee. Maintain a tall and proper posture. Lean into front leg to feel a stretch down your hip and quadriceps. Pulse for three counts and then hold in a stretched position for ten seconds. Repeat five times on each side.

Belly button squeezes. Try this both standing up and sitting. While maintaining a full and natural breath, draw your belly button in toward your spine and feel your inner abdominal muscles tighten. Once you can do this and maintain strength and breathing, you can try raising one foot off the ground (sitting or standing) while maintaining the pulled in navel. You will strengthen inner core muscles that are important for spinal stability and protection.

A HEALTHY BACK

In 2001, the Bureau of Labor Statistics reported 372,683 back injury cases involving days away from work.. The estimated annual cost for back pain is $20 billion to $50 billion and results in approximately 149 million lost workdays per year. This is significant to the work system and to your everyday health. The annual productivity losses resulting from lost workdays are estimated to be $28 billion.

What can you do to prevent or lessen your chances of obtaining a low back injury in your lifetime? Should you wear a lifting belt at the gym, be sedentary because that hurts less, or buy a back brace? The answer is no to all of the previous options.

The best option for low back health is appropriate and adequate exercises. If you are currently experiencing low back pain, you should rule out any major injuries such as a herniated disc by seeing your medical provider first.

The greatest risk people take is having a weak core and then loading the spine with a heavy weight and jerking it around (for example, imagine picking up a giant box at Costco after shopping and throwing your back out). How do we get such weak cores? Well, the first problem lies in our sedentary lifestyles. Sitting at a computer, in the car, or at work can reduce your back's need to stabilize your posture. We tend to slouch and let our trunks relax.

Also, excess weight gain in the abdomen can increase the curve in the low back and cause for an abnormal force distribution throughout the spine.

People also tend to do the wrong type of strengthening moves and focus heavily on their abdominals (rectus abdominus), which only aids in flexing the spine (bending forward). However, our core muscles actually include our deep corset muscle (the transverse abdominus), external and internal obliques, quadratus lumborum, hip flexors, gluteal muscles, and spinal erectors. It takes a balance of these muscles to enable us to move appropriately throughout our daily lives and prevent major injury.

Lastly, posture is very important as it helps train our spine in what proper alignment feels like. Proper posture will help prevent you from positioning yourself in dangerous ways.

Before trying the following activities, try standing up nice and tall with shoulders over your hips and hips over your heels with slightly relaxed, not locked out knees. Make sure to also pull your chin back and rotate your palms out before relaxing them; this helps pull your shoulders back where they belong. Now, pull in your belly button as far back as you can toward your spine. This occurs because of contraction of your transverse abdominus, which is that corset muscle that pulls everything inward. This muscle helps support your back and should be contracted before lifting anything.

Perform the following exercise for ten repetitions, three times a week.

Pilates Roll-Up

Lying flat, legs extended, arms over shoulders and pulling your belly button in, slowly inhale. On the exhale, curl your body up as you push each vertebrae of your spine into the ground. Continue to roll up and suck in the belly to reach out toward or over your toes. The objective is not to flatten your belly to your legs, but to pull your belly in and over your lap as you reach forward. Slowly lower down with legs extended and toes flexed. Make sure you lower one vertebra at a time. Repeat.

Combination Plank

Face down on your elbows and toes; pull your belly button up and in. Make sure your hips are parallel to your shoulders before starting. Pull your right knee into your chest but maintain a flat back, then straighten and extend your right foot back and extend at the hip. As you extend that foot up, do not arch your lower back. Now try with your left leg; repeat back and forth.

Ball Back Extension

Lay on your back over an exercise ball with legs extended and the ball under your hips. With your hands behind your head and neck relaxed, slowly raise your back up but still contract your abdominals and pull your navel in so your stomach is not relaxed. Slowly lower back down and repeat.

Tips:

- You can buy an exercise ball at any sporting goods store. You can use it for exercises and use it to sit on at your desk instead of a chair. This will help you maintain better posture.

- Practice pulling your navel in while you are driving, sitting at your computer, or watching television. This helps train your abdominals to stay contracted and conditions them to have better endurance.

- If you sit at a desk all day, try not to cross your legs. Instead, place your feet up on a slight inclined step and sit up nice and tall. Crossing your legs can put your spine off balance and cause problems down the road.

- Get up and do some squats and stretch your hip flexors. You might wonder what squats will do to help your back, but sitting all day relaxes your glutes and tightens your hip flexors. So every few hours, stand up and do ten squats and then lunge with each foot forward for thirty seconds to stretch your opposite hamstring!

Perhaps you already experience back pain. No matter what caused your back injury, the pain can sideline you from a normal workout and even your normal daily life! Before starting any exercise routine, you should be cleared by your supervising physician and/or physical therapist. Often, the first thing you will get back to is walking. Seated exercises, like cycling, can actually place more unnecessary stress on your vertebrae and spinal column, which could exacerbate your pain. So it might be more comfortable for you to hit the treadmill or walk outdoors before sitting on a bicycle, for example. Increase your speed slowly to protect your back from spasming into pain.

Weight training is definitely an important portion of your workout and should be slowly incorporated back into your exercise routine. One of the biggest mistakes that people make after a back injury is to stop all strength training and core work because they are fearful they will hurt their back again. Taking too much time away from strengthening exercises can increase your risk of further hurting your back because your stabilization and core muscles will be weaker. To ease back into weight lifting, you need to first be sure that your back is pain free and rehabilitated. After doing rehabilitation to strengthen your deep core muscles (transverse abdominus, obliques, and quadratus lumborum), you can start to ease back into full body lifts.

The risk with weight training and back injuries begin with the form and posture in which you lift. Your back should have normal curves to it. It should curve in (concave) at your lower (lumbar) spine and cervical (neck) regions. The middle portion (thoracic) should cave out (convex). When you lift weights (or daily objects that are heavy), focus on maintaining this normal S-shape curvature of your spine. Do not try to flatten or arch your back while performing any lift. Maintain the normal curve throughout the entire range.

The way to maintain back stabilization and strength during a resistance move is to focus on tightening the entire area. A good way to stabilize your back is to concentrate on "zipping up" your front side and sucking your belly button in toward your spine. By performing a kegel exercise (contracting the muscles of the pelvic floor), you can increase the tightening of the muscles that surround and protect your low back. Pulling in your navel improves the tightening of the transverse abdominus to stabilize the spine and narrow your waist. If you stray away from contracting your entire core and maintaining your normal curvature, you risk hurting your back again.

As well, try to avoid lifting weight (dumbbells or a heavy grocery bag) while twisting your spine. If you have diagnosed disc herniation or the possibility of disc abnormalities, you could cause severe damage with rotational moves and with hyperextension moves.

If contracting all of these muscles feels confusing and difficult, practice during your normal, everyday activities such as when you are driving in the car or sitting at the computer. It helps to practice contracting and pulling in your core so that it translates to better core control during weight room mechanics.

INJURIES FROM OVER-EXERCISING

We often hear about people not exercising enough. Sedentary lifestyle is one of the leading risks of obesity and possibly heart disease; there is much evidence to suggest that exercise helps prevent disease and improve health. However, it is possible for a person to exercise too much and possibly harm their health.

Too much of a good thing is something that many Americans tend to do. For example, taking a multivitamin might help improve your health but taking multiple bottles of various supplements can have harmful effects if they interact or you overdose on various vitamins. The biggest risk to exercising too much and too intensely is the lack of recovery. The body needs adequate time to repair and regenerate fibers and connective tissue that have been damaged during intense exercise. As well, free radical formation is increased with high intensity exercise and could cause damage to tissue.

Some research has found possible evidence of severe effects of excessive exercise. A study published in the Journal of Applied Physiology, found that older men who trained most of their lives at a strenuous level had higher levels of fibrosis of their hearts (hardening or scar tissue of the heart muscle).

The Journal of Applied Physiology's February 2011 study concluded that an unexpectedly high prevalence (50 percent) of myocardial fibrosis was observed in healthy, asymptomatic life-long veteran male athletes, compared to zero cases in age-matched veteran controls and young athletes. This data suggests a link between life-long endurance exercise and myocardial fibrosis that requires further investigation. The New York Times recently reported on a 2008 German study that found that older marathon runners had higher levels of fibrosis of the heart. Other causes of fibrosis could be present but it does bring question to the possibility of a maximum threshold for training, moving from health effects to harmful effects.

When you are trying to lose weight or improve muscular or cardiovascular strength, you must push yourself into overload. Overload is increasing the demand on the physiological processes of your body to elicit a response. In terms of cardiovascular response, if the goal was increased endurance then you could train by running, performing intervals, or hill repeats. For increased strength, you might lift heavier weights or change the exercises. When you are putting yourself in an overload situation, you will get positive results. However, if you continue to push beyond overload, you will end up overtraining. Overtraining can cause muscle fatigue, injury, lack of sleep, and weight loss. Pushing the body enough to see a positive effect—while minimizing overtraining—is a constant evaluation process. To prevent overtraining, it is recommended to have at least one day of rest a week. Your rest day can be complete rest from exercise or include light, active rest such as walking the dog.

Varying the training intensity is also necessary. Running could be more intense for a couple days in the week while others are less intense. For example, Mondays could be for hill training and Wednesdays for interval training. On another day, running could be performed at a lower intensity for enjoyment; this could be a longer, slower run. Other days should include cross-training activities such as swimming or cycling. Too much of one activity, especially high-impact running, can cause increased risk for injury. Some well-conditioned runners can run more frequently than others without injury, but it is still recommended that some days be lighter in intensity.

Any sport or training routine should include enjoyment and excitement about the journey. If you or someone you know has moved from excitement to frustration and obsession with a certain exercise behavior, this could be a red flag that they need some time off.

CHAPTER 8

PREVENTING AND MANAGING ILLNESSES

I t is easy to let chronic disease and unrelenting physical conditions keep you from getting the best of your workout routine. Instead of sidelining exercise altogether, you can accommodate your training program with the various conditions you might incur and still get great results. About 25.8 million people in the United States, or 8.3 percent of the population, have diabetes and 10.5 percent (30.2 million) of the US population has been diagnosed with asthma in their lifetime! Many of us are struggling against ailments that make it difficult to exercise. Here are some ways to make the most of your workout while working with the conditions you have.

DIABETES

For diabetics, one of the best ways to lessen symptoms and physical hardship is through regular exercise. The American College of Sports Medicine recommends a minimum of 150 minutes per week of moderate-to-vigorous aerobic exercise spread out at least three days during the week, with no more than two consecutive days between bouts of aerobic activity. Resistance exercise (strength training) could be as important as aerobic training in diabetes management. Exercise can improve glucose (blood sugar) uptake by the cells, therefore increasing insulin sensitivity. Much research shows that even exercising once a week improves blood glucose levels and insulin sensitivity.

Tips:

- Get supervision: Exercise intervention studies showing the greatest effect on blood sugar control have all involved supervision of exercise sessions by qualified exercise trainers. At least in the beginning, have a trained professional supervise your workouts for safety and effectiveness. Try hiring a trainer for just a couple sessions or join a group exercise class.

- Prevent hypoglycemia: If you're not insulin dependent, your risk of hypoglycemia is less. However, try to monitor blood glucose before and after exercise and supplement with a carbohydrate snack if needed.

- Be aware of medications: If you are finding that hypoglycemia is more common after a bout of exercise you might want to talk to your physician about decreasing insulin and/or drug treatment. If you're on beta-blockers, you might not see an elevated heart rate response to exercise so don't push yourself too hard in a group exercise format if they are monitoring heart rate.

- If you are accustomed to exercise, try increasing activity to vigorous if your physician approves.

- Watch those feet: Long term diabetes can lead to peripheral artery disease and a loss of sensation in the lower extremities. Wear good footwear and be aware of any changes in circulation or loss of balance.

- Perform large muscle group exercise. Instead of doing isolated weight training, such as weight machines, try water aerobics, dance class, seated bicycling, or walking.

- Retinopathy, or macular degeneration, is common in diabetics. Make sure you avoid high intensity exercise or heavy resistance training. Instead, try low-intensity weights and lower intensity aerobics like walking for exercise.

- Daily movement is more important than an organized bout of exercise in a gym. Get moving! Physical activity will help control blood sugar levels and is something you can stick to. Put on your tennis shoes and go for a nice walk!

ASTHMA

Asthma affects approximately 20 million Americans. During an asthma attack, muscles around the airways tighten up, making the airways narrower so less air flows through. Common symptoms of asthma include coughing, wheezing, difficulty breathing, and chest tightness.

Asthma is a common deterrent to exercise. This can often cause a person to worsen in symptoms and health as they neglect physical activity in fear of asthmatic attacks. Studies like the ones published in the Journal of Asthma in 2006 report that asthmatic patients pre-dispose themselves to long-term health risks from lack of activity. It is important that asthmatics still have adequate physical activity. Knowing how to prepare and what types of activities to perform can help lessen symptoms and improve health. Asthmatics tend to have lower forced expiratory volumes (FEV), which is the volume of air exhaled in the first second of forced exhalation starting from full inspiration. Other respiratory conditions with extremely restricted FEV are those who suffer from chronic obstructive pulmonary disease (COPD).

One of the most risky environments for an asthmatic to exercise is in a cold and dry environment. When the air is cold and dry, the bronchial airways are constricted and cause higher resistance to airflow. Our airways naturally moisten the air we breathe but when you are breathing heavily in a dry environment the bronchial airways become dry and can trigger an asthmatic reaction. When your ventilation, or breathing rate, increases, this can also cause far more asthmatic symptoms such as airway tightening and constriction. For those with exercise-induced asthma, their symptoms usually peak at eight to fifteen minutes after exercise begins and can last up to three hours after exercise ceases.

A study performed at the University of Washington (2000) on asthmatic patients found that mild aerobic conditioning improved FEV and increased VO2 (used to measure cardio respiratory fitness). The patients exercised for ten weeks, performing step aerobics three times a week. They maintained their intensity to 70 percent the VO2max, which would be equivalent to a seven on a one to ten rate of perceived exertion scale. So they felt that they were working hard but were in control of their breathing at this intensity. The study found that this level of conditioning, with the aid of β-agonist drugs such as albuterol, allows for improved aerobic function without extreme events. In fact, in this study it was found that the onset of shortness of breath for asthma patients' was delayed with chronic exercise training. So by the end of the ten-week program they could exercise at a higher intensity than prior to the training without any shortness of breath.

Therefore, asthmatic patients can and should exercise to increase their aerobic capacity. Continued exercise can also lessen the symptoms and onset of asthma attacks from and during exercise. Asthma patients should have a lengthened warm-up to their exercise session, lasting up to ten minutes. Taking a bronchodilator prior to exercise can help lessen symptoms such as tightened airways.

Running and jogging type activities can also trigger asthma attacks due to their more vigorous nature. Therefore, it is wise to try things such as swimming and yoga first while getting your asthma in control and still getting aerobic conditioning. Swimming is good because you are in a warm and humid environment, which can help your symptoms. Most importantly, work up gradually. It is important that you start slowly at an activity that does not cause shortness of breath. Work up your intensity and then continue to try new activities at a low intensity.

The American College of Sports Medicine recommends these tips for asthmatic exercisers:

- Consult with an allergist and/or immunologist prior to starting an exercise program. The physician may test you to determine what you are allergic to and to possibly diagnose asthma. The doctor can then effectively treat the symptoms and recommend activities to do and to avoid.

- Take all allergy and asthma medications as prescribed.
- Breathe through the nose as much as possible when exercising. The nasal passages act as natural filters and humidifiers to maintain air at proper temperatures as well as filter out allergens, pollutants, and irritants.
- Exercise indoors during extreme temperatures and when allergen counts are high; pollen counts are usually highest in the morning and increase again in the afternoon.
- When exercising indoors, keep windows and doors closed to reduce allergen exposure; try to exercise on mats rather than carpeting.
- When exercising outdoors, avoid areas that contain high concentrations of allergens and irritants (e.g., fields, trees, busy roads, factories).
- Always have your asthma rescue medication on hand when exercising. You may be instructed to take your medication shortly before exercise; use as prescribed by your physician.
- Perform a prolonged aerobic warm-up and cool-down (fifteen minutes each) if you have asthma; this can

reduce the chances or severity of exercise-induced asthma.

- Postpone exercise if asthma symptoms are not well-controlled of if you have a cold or respiratory infection.

MANAGING STRESS

Stress is a very natural part of being human. Stress is the component that allows us to react quickly to life or death situations. This "fight or flight" mechanism allowed our ancestors to run away from a wild animal and to also catch that prey for dinner. Therefore, stress is a completely natural part of human behavior and is actually good for survival.

However, we have to realize how stress affects us in today's world. The type of stress we burden now is a constant dose of the stresses of life. When you are under stress (imagine running away from a wild bull), your body releases extra doses of epinephrine (adrenaline), norepinephrine, and cortisol (a stress hormone), which increases your blood pressure, blood flow, and increases glucose levels to allow you to react at a quicker pace and for a longer period of time. This surge of hormones can increase your heart and immune function. In fact, some research shows that certain levels of stress can decrease your risk for Alzheimer's and other neurological disorders from an increased brain capacity and blood flow. The problem arises when this increased level of hormones lasts longer and longer in our everyday lives. Your body is not supposed to have a continual onslaught of increased adrenaline and cortisol running through it. An increased level of these hormones on an ongoing basis will cause your body to kick into overdrive in a negative way.

This long-term stress state is called chronic stress. Many Americans suffer from chronic stress. The problem arises when we do not have a place to release our stress. Our stress begins to creep into every facet of our lives. For example, instead of leaving stress at work, we bring it home and live under a constant state of anxiety and a revved up emotional state. It is as if we cannot "let it go." Weeks of increased stress keep your blood pressure and resting heart rate elevated which can lead to heart function problems and cardiovascular risk.

If you are continually stressed, you will lose sleep, which can cause fatigue and depression. Depression is even more common if you feel that your stress is out of your control. Studies have shown that those who feel in control of their stressors tend to have less depression and get out of the chronic stress cycle more easily. Other long-term effects of stress include a risk for obesity. High levels of cortisol have shown to increase abdominal obesity, which is a marker for increased risk for heart disease. So, although cortisol can help you improve physical performance, long-term high levels can increase the risk for obesity.

A few signs that your physical body is suffering from stress are these symptoms: mental unclarity, depression, insomnia, frequent colds, inflammatory bowels, and irritability. If you feel that you have chronic stress, then work on finding a solution for dealing with the stress. It is nearly impossible to completely get rid of stress in your life, especially with today's economy and international uneasiness. Instead of trying to eliminate stress, find a way to release it. There are many common avenues you can take to lessen the physical impact of stress on your body.

If you are having a hard time falling asleep at night then make sure you have a relaxing bedtime ritual. Give yourself at least fifteen minutes to allow the body and brain to slow down. Begin your routine once the house has quieted down. First write down anything that is still swarming in your head. Then take a lukewarm, not hot shower. A hot shower can often lengthen the time to sleep since your body has to work at cooling the core temperature down. After getting out of the shower, stretch your major muscle groups in a dark and quiet place for at least five minutes, holding each stretch for a minimum of thirty seconds. The most important thing you can do is take deep breaths to increase oxygenation and slow your heart rate. Then lie down in a dark and quiet room.

If you feel highly stressed during your day, then step away from your desk or step outside and take ten deep, long inhales and exhales. You can even stretch while breathing to improve relaxation.

Yoga is another popular way to relieve stress. And although yoga has become a very fashionable and popular thing to do, the science behind it is pretty amazing. In hatha yoga, where breathing is key, you learn to control your breathing pattern and even slow your heart rate. The combination of physical exertion, mental clarity, and deep breathing teaches your nervous system how to breathe deeply even when your body is under exertion. This pattern can help you breathe deeper during the day and under stressful situations, therefore improving your physical health when stress hits.

Remember that chronic stress is bad for your physical wellbeing but that stress can be healthy. Stress can motivate you to work towards a goal; it can drive you to work harder and also strengthen your body for the future. However, learn to deal with high levels of chronic stress to decrease your risk for obesity, heart disease, and neurological problems.

MASSAGE

Massage is moving from a luxury to an essential component in many people's lives. Many people receive massage therapy for the first time as treatment for an injury or accident. Others receive massage as a treat celebrating a special occasion. No matter how you have experienced massage, you are more than likely looking forward to your next appointment!

There are three major forms of massage therapy. The main one most people know about is massage. Massage is defined as the application of soft tissue and muscular manipulation techniques to the body. Bodywork is another that involves manipulation, movement, and repatterning that causes structural change to the body. Another form is called somatic in which a whole-body approach is used. These are just a few. There are over 250 different specialty types of massage therapy. Many massage therapists use a variety of these forms during one massage session or throughout their session depending on their particular clients' needs.

Is massage and bodywork considered medicinal or physically beneficial to your body? The Associate Bodywork and Massage Professional Association list many benefits to massage therapy.

It can alleviate low back pain, stretch tense or weak muscles, help muscle recovery after an intense workout, improve flexibility, reduce scar tissue formation, improve circulation by increasing blood and nutrient flow to tissues, and reduce post surgery adhesions and swelling. Other physical benefits of massage include relieving migraine pain from releasing tension that is exacerbating the problem, improving the condition of the body's largest organ, the skin, and improving immunity by increasing lymph circulation. Massage can also release endorphins that are the body's natural painkillers, resulting in a euphoric sense of wellbeing.

Massage is also wonderful for expectant and recovering mothers. It lessens muscle spasm and stiffness, thus allowing for easier labor and quicker recovery.

One of the greatest benefits of massage is the mental and emotional factor. Many health professionals agree that upwards of 90 percent of all disease is somehow linked to stress. Massage can alleviate stress by improving your sleep, decreasing anxiety, giving you greater energy throughout the day, improving concentration and circulation to your brain, as well as reducing fatigue. During a massage, you are allowed a break from it all. It is very rare for any of us to take some time apart from our busy lives and relax. We often go ninety miles an hour and then fall in to bed with our mind racing with the day's stress.

Massage decreases arthritic pain and joint stiffness. Asthmatics can improve their pulmonary circulation and airflow from massage therapy. Cardiac patients have shown a decrease in systolic blood pressure, anxiety, and stress hormones. For many women, massage has also shown to decrease menstrual cycle pain and cramping.

Massage has become an integral part of many athletes and every-day people's physical regimen. Regular appointments with a massage therapist can help you stay on top of muscle imbalances, tightness, and scar tissue. A qualified massage therapist should be able to help you determine muscle imbalances and how to improve your physical health. Many health professionals can offer a referral to you if you have a particular need.

It is very important for you to make sure you are getting a massage from a licensed massage therapist. The website www.massagetherapy.com allows you to pick from many various forms of massage and where they are located. You can choose from Swedish massage, shiatsu, therapeutic, and even infant touch massage. There are endless options on this website; it also allows you to make sure your massage professional is licensed in their specialty.

Do not for one second feel guilty about massage. It is a technique that has been used for thousands of years to benefit the body and help it heal. Keep this technique and practice as part of your wellbeing routine.

PERIPHERAL ARTERIAL DISEASE

If you notice burning in your calves while you are exercising, consider the source. Pain and burning in your lower calves could be caused from a number of issues. The first and least serious cause could be from a lack of warming up and possibly too tight lower leg muscles. If you are not used to working out and have just begun a program, you might be experiencing leg cramping as you become fatigued. As well, tightly tied shoelaces can cause decreased blood circulation, with increased tingling and a numbness sensation. But if you are wearing new shoes with appropriate insoles and attire then you might have other deeper issues.

Burning sensation in the calves can sometimes be a sign of peripheral arterial disease (PAD). PAD is a common but serious chronic condition that can increase your risk of a heart attack or stroke. So what is PAD? PAD is systemic (not around your heart but in your extremities) atherosclerosis (narrowing of arteries from plaque deposits). In the January/February 2010 edition of ACSM's Health and Fitness Journal, the authors report that PAD affects one in twenty people in Americans who are over the age of fifty. And many of those who have PAD go undiagnosed and live with the symptoms. High cholesterol, hypertension (high blood pressure), and cigarette smoking are all precursors and often go along with PAD.

Cramping is often most evident in the calves but is also seen in the thighs. Due to narrowing of the systemic arteries, not enough blood—and therefore oxygen—is being delivered to the tissues that are working so hard. Increasing pain often causes people to sit down and rest and this can alleviate pain for the short term.

Researchers in the ACSM journal report that exercise can help prevent and lessen the symptoms and pain associated with PAD. If you think you might have signs of PAD, you should consult your physician. Exercise should include walking on the treadmill or outside for at least thirty to sixty minutes. But if you have pain when you begin, then you should slowly progress to this duration. You might want to walk a few times throughout the day and build up to thirty minutes all at once. Make sure you allow rest between bouts of exercise.

Begin your walk with a slow pace to increase blood flow. If you feel pain while walking, you could continue walking until you reach a pain scale of three. The PAD pain scale goes from zero to four with zero being no pain to four being maximal pain. Try to walk three to five times a week.

Resistance training has also shown to improve PAD. Aim to perform resistance training two to three days a week, performing eight to ten multi-joint exercises for each major muscle group. Complete eight to fifteen repetitions of each exercise and two to four sets of each. For people with PAD, whole body exercises might be the most beneficial!

Continued exercise can improve your symptoms and lessen the chance of PAD progressing. Exercise will also help improve your cholesterol and lower your chance of heart attack and stroke. However, if you continue to have pain during most or all of your activity, then consult your physician.

SEASONAL ALLERGIES

An allergic reaction occurs when your body's immune system reacts to fend off any foreign substance. Normally your body's response systems would only be fired up if you were invaded by some type of bacteria or virus that warranted sufficient harm. But for some people, pollen and other substances in the air (pollution, grass, etc.) or foods you ingest can trigger the same immune response. Your immune system causes a release of histamines that cause a runny nose, itchy eyes, and scratchy throat.

What makes the reaction much worse at some times of the year is stagnant and warm air. Oftentimes, weather with poor air quality and circulation can worsen the pollens' effects on your body.

Before recommending a particular regimen, it is highly important that you see a physician to rule out any major pulmonary or asthmatic problem.

If you are suffering from allergies it can be tempting to avoid exercise all together but it is recommended to work around some of your difficulties to continue what is good for your heart and body. It can help a person to breathe through their nose instead of their mouth because their nose can act as a filter, preventing some allergens to get deep within the body and minimizing the cascade of reactions. Exercising very late in the day can help your reactions. Pollen counts are usually highest in the mornings and are the least in wet, chilly evenings, which could lessen your allergic reaction.

If you are fairly sure you have allergies, you can see your physician to be tested from a particular allergy. If you believe you are allergic to ragweed pollen, which can travel hundreds of miles, then you might want to stay away from wooded areas and areas near open fields full of ragweed. Instead, opt for a paved path near some water that will have less ragweed and some fresh air movement.

Warm up for at least ten minutes to allow your lungs and bronchial tubes to warm up and prevent constriction. You also want to be very cautious of any unwanted symptoms and stop if you feel faint or have trouble breathing.

Fewer allergy symptoms are also seen in sports with short bursts of activity versus long duration activities. So opt for interval training over long distance runs.

If you are suffering from a severe cold or congestion then wait to exercise until you are symptom free. Sever congestion can prevent the filtration from happening in your nasal passages.

You can also try to cover your nose and mouth with a handkerchief. This can help warm and humidify the air before it reaches your bronchioles, which lessens any constriction of your airways. It can also help filter some of the pollen.

If you continue to experience severe discomfort as bronchospasms cause difficulty breathing, exercise indoors where there is sufficient air filtration.

When stretching at the gym, make sure you use a mat since many allergens lurk on the carpets.

If your allergies are severe, then carry an Epi-pen for emergencies and carry proper medical identification. Your doctor might also prescribe an inhaler for prevention and treatment.

Although summer weather is conducive to exercising outdoors, summer can be the worst time of year to be outdoors for those with allergies. Check the website www.pollen.com you can find your local pollen count forecast. The great thing about www.pollen.com is that you can have a pollen forecast emailed directly to you on a regular basis so you are aware of the dangers for you.

DECREASING RISK OF ILLNESS

Exercise can be one of the most effective ways of decreasing your risk for sickness and disease. Even a few minutes of exercise each day can be extremely helpful to your immune system.

Every time you exercise, your body's immune system is heightened and improved. As well, when you exercise, you sleep better and that could help boost your immune system. Researchers in immunology give some reasons to why exercise could help your immunity. Exercise could help flush bacteria out of your lungs. Exercise sends more white blood cells and antibodies throughout your body, fighting off any bacterial infections present. Exercise could also increase your body temperature enough that it kills off bacteria; much like a fever does when you get sick. Exercise can also decrease the release of stress hormones, which often increase the likelihood of illness.

It is very important that you remember that more isn't always better. There are some studies published by the

National Institutes of Health on the increased occurrence of upper respiratory infections (UPRI) by those who perform intense exercise for extreme minutes/hours a week. For example, extreme cardiovascular endurance athletes tend to have higher rates of upper respiratory infections than those who exercise at a moderate level. So exercise smart and do not overdo it. Moderate exercise on a regular basis will help your immunity the best!

PHYSICAL ACTIVITY

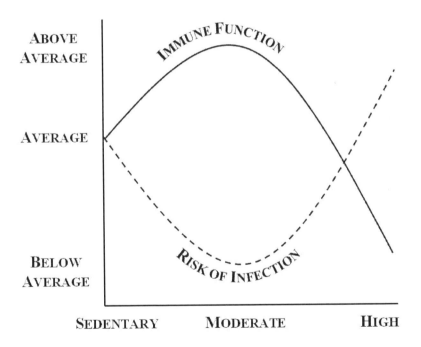

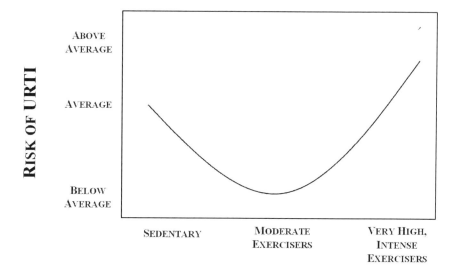

AMOUNT AND INTENSITY OF EXERCISE

When NOT to exercise:

You should try to remember this:

- If your symptoms are from the neck up, you are usually okay to go out for a low- to moderate intensity workout such as a brisk walk or slow jog. This can often clear your congestion and give you renewed energy. However if your symptoms are below the neck (extreme sore throat with severe chest congestion and bad cough), you should take the day off. Maybe a trip to the doctor to have your lungs listened to or heard is a good idea.

- If you risk infecting others such as in a closed, poorly ventilated area or in a pool, you should stay home! You do not want to spread a virus or bacteria; if you are going to exercise, try going out for a nice walk on your own!

EXERCISING IN THE COLD

Do you remember hearing from your mother as a child, "Wear a jacket, it's cold outside and you don't want to get sick"? I think we have all heard that or have said that in our lives. However, that is just a myth. The presence of bacteria and viruses are what cause illness. So if you have already been infected with the bacteria, it probably doesn't matter if you are cold or not.

To safeguard yourself from illness, wash your hands, get ample amounts of sleep, eat a healthy diet, and stay away from those who are contagious. It usually takes a few days for an illness to present symptoms (the incubation period).

Bundling up can help you better regulate body temperature so it is a good idea to follow the "what to wear" guidelines.

What to wear when exercising in cold weather

If you are going to be out exercising in cold weather, then:

- Wear layers. It will be easy to take off one layer at a time when you start to warm up.

- Cover up your ears if they are sensitive to the cold.

- Wear fabric that wicks moisture away from your skin.

- Take some water and food with you if you are going to be gone for a while. The cold might slow you down and you want to be prepared.

- Tell someone where you are headed. It is always smart to give someone your route.

- Watch out for slick spots, both for you and for any cars driving by if you are out on the roads.

CHAPTER 9

CHILDHOOD HEALTH

Our nation's next generation is at risk of possibly dying before their parents if health statistics and obesity rates are not improved. The Center of Disease and Control reports that childhood obesity has more than doubled in children and quadrupled in adolescents in the past 30 years. The percentage of children aged 6-11 years in the United States who were obese increased from 7% in 1980 to nearly 18% in 2012. Similarly, the percentage of adolescents aged 12-19 years who were obese increased from 5% to nearly 21% over the same period of 30 years. And in 2012, more than one third of children and adolescents were overweight or obese. Children are growing up in a society that requires very little physical activity on a regular basis and provides them a plethora of convenient food choices. Kids are going home from school to empty houses and are often told to stay inside where it is safer and therefore get much less physical activity. Food of convenience are becoming the norm for many children whose families are too busy to prepare family meals and children are increasing their size as a result in a culture shift. Technology, unhealthy good-tasting food, and a lack of activity has increased the childhood obesity prevalence and has caused small children to suffer from high blood pressure and type 2 diabetes.

EXERCISING IN PREGNANCY

Your child's health begins while he or she is unborn.
Then again, if you don't plan to have another child, you can
skip to page 265.

Historically, there was an era when pregnant women were warned not to exercise in order to protect the baby and due to fear of causing a miscarriage or fetal damage. However, research and continued education has led to changed recommendations. The American Congress of Obstetricians and Gynecologists (ACOG) encourage physical activity during pregnancy for women who were previously active. For those who were not, they should seek physician approval and guidance to begin an exercise program. The ACOG recommends that pregnant women be physical active at least thirty minutes a day, most days of the week.

The benefits of exercise include: reduced back pain, constipation, and bloating; prevention of gestational diabetes; increased energy; improved mood and posture; the promotion of muscle tone, strength, and endurance; improved sleep; and improved labor and delivery.

One of the greatest reasons for prenatal exercise is to prevent and manage gestational diabetes. The American Diabetes Association has endorsed exercise as helpful adjunctive therapy for gestational diabetes when altering the diet alone is not sufficient. Exercise can also help the mother feel more physically fit to deal with the stress of childbirth and recovery. After the birth, exercise will help her return to her healthy pre-pregnancy weight much sooner.

Along with the Center for Disease Control and the American College of Sports Medicine, the ACOG recommends that pregnant women accumulate at least thirty minutes most days of sustained cardiovascular activity that requires a rate of perceived exertion between 12-14 on a scale of 6-20 (called the Borg Scale). The mode of exercise should include those that are rhythmic in nature such as swimming, cycling, and walking. Flexibility and resistance exercises should also be performed. Resistance training should be done twice a week with lower intensity, lower weight, and higher repetitions. Studies have found that lower intensity weight training does not alter fetal heart rates.

Pregnancy Exercise Concerns

Your body is different when pregnant, mostly due to hormone and bodily changes. When you are pregnant, hormones that allow your ligaments to stretch for accommodating the fetus and delivery also increase the laxity of your other joints. So you might feel some uncomfortable pulls while exercising. Be careful and listen to your body. Also, make sure to wear supportive clothing, such as a comfortable sports bra and shoes. Stay hydrated before, during, and after exercise. Try to avoid exercising in the heat of the day, as overheating is a big concern for pregnant women. Lastly, a growing belly can throw your center of gravity off and increase your risk for falling and injury so make sure to exercise on level terrain and watch your step.

As the pregnancy progresses, loading the spine with weight should be avoided or done with caution to prevent lower back injury. The increased weight of the baby and higher levels of hormones cause the back to have an increased lordortic (arched) curve and could increase the risk for injury.

Exercise lying flat on the back or lying on the stomach should be avoided after the first trimester. If you want to continue doing exercises like a dumbbell bench press then you might be able to continue doing them on an incline bench where you are sitting more upright.

Extreme athletics that involve contact and possible injury such as basketball, soccer, hockey, and even rock climbing pose a severe risk to the fetus and mother. Exercising at higher elevation is also risky for those who are not acclimated to it. Environmental factors such as heat also play a role. To prevent dehydration and a rise in body temperature, a pregnant woman should exercise in a well-ventilated, air-conditioned room if the weather is warm outdoors.

Proper hydration while exercising is imperative. It is very important the mother stay hydrated at all times by carrying water with her and taking small sips throughout the workout. Adequately warming up and cooling down is also important to regulate blood pressure and improve warming up of musculature to prevent injury.

Pregnancy is not the time to start an intense exercise program or train for a competitive sport. However, it is the perfect time to enjoy your exercise program and focus on holistic wellness that incorporates activities such as walking, swimming, and yoga. If you are already a competitive athlete, you can still maintain much of your fitness but be careful to listen to your body. Remember that you are building another human being—that is your body's priority.

When to Stop Exercise

If you encounter any of the following symptoms, you should stop exercising and consult your physician:

- Dizziness or faint feeling

- Vaginal bleeding

- Headache

- Chest pain

- Shortness of breath

- Fluid leakage

- Abdominal pain or contractions

- Calf pain or swelling

- Reduced fetal movement

Best Pregnancy Exercises

Kegels: The most effective way to perform kegels is to squat down with feet wide and knees in line with toes. Slowly contract the pelvic floor (it will feel like you are stopping the flow of urine) and hold for at least ten seconds or more. Then slowly release the contraction and repeat fifty to one hundred times. Kegels will help during delivery, give you flexibility, and speed up your childbirth recovery.

Walking: Just thirty minutes of walking can make you feel energized and more flexible.

Wide leg bodyweight squats: Avoid putting weights on your back once you are in the second trimester. Place your feet wider than hip-width, point toes out slightly, and keep your knees aligned with your toes. Slowly lower down into a squat while maintaining a stable spine. Hold for two seconds at the bottom (just about 90 degrees), and slowly return to standing. Repeat fifteen times.

Modified yoga Sun Salutations:

1. Stand with your feet mat-width apart, inhale with arms extended overhead.
2. Exhale. Bend the knees as you come down to Camper's Pose, keeping the feet wide and parallel.
3. Inhale. Bring the palms flat inside the feet, and step the right leg back to a lunge.
4. Exhale. Step the left foot back to Downward Facing Dog.
5. Inhale. Come forward to a Plank position.
6. Exhale. Drop the knees to the floor, and bend the elbows straight back as in Chaturanga Dandasana.
7. Exhale. Push back to Downward Facing Dog.
8. Inhale. Bring the right foot forward to the outside of the right foot coming into a Lunge.
9. Exhale. Step the left foot to the outside of the left hand coming into Camper's Pose.
10. Go back to the start with arms overhead, feet mat-width apart. Repeat sequence.

EASY AND HEALTHY SCHOOL MEALS

When summer comes to a close and school is about to begin, getting all of your children's school supplies and clothes are usually the most important things on your mind. Thinking about breakfasts and lunches on school days can feel cumbersome but what your children eat is one of the most important aspects to their day. Without a healthy breakfast and lunch, your child will not be as alert and efficient in the classroom or after-school activity. With children who dread that morning alarm, it can feel even more challenging to get them a healthy breakfast before they whisk out the door.

One of the best things you can do for your child is feed them healthy food. And the most important meal of the day is breakfast. Have healthy food on hand and then they have healthy options. It helps if you eat the healthy foods you want them to eat so they are not being asked to eat something different than the rest of the family.

Aim for a mix of complex carbohydrates, protein, and healthy fats. Complex carbohydrates include things like oatmeal, whole grain cereal, or whole-wheat English muffins. Try low-sugar versions of instant oatmeal for a tasty but quick whole grain option. To make sure you are getting a whole grain cereal, check the label. It should have a high level of fiber; anything above five grams per serving is sufficient. Also look to see that the sugar content is low. Too much sugar in the morning can lead to a mental and physical crash early in the morning.

Great protein options are eggs, non-fat yogurt, or cottage cheese. Although eggs have been given a bad reputation, they are a good source of protein and do not increase cholesterol in normal subjects if eaten moderately.

Great sources of healthy fat are all natural peanut butter and ground flaxseed (can be added to your cereal). You can also sprinkle almonds or walnuts on your cold or hot cereal. It only takes five or ten minutes to prepare a healthy breakfast. That short amount of time could make a giant impact on how focused your child will be in the classroom.

Lunch is a meal where you are not present to watch that they eat what you pack, but it is your responsibility to prepare them with a healthy meal option. Unfortunately, a school provided lunch is often not the healthiest option. They are inexpensive and are now offering more healthy alternatives than they used to, however, most children will choose the unhealthy options such as pizza and hamburgers. Try to help your child pack his or her lunch the night before. Involve them in the process so that they like what they will be eating. Discuss with your kids your desire for them to like their lunch but that eating unhealthy and high-fat foods will decrease their performance and make them feel sluggish.

You can make the lunch taste good while keeping it full of color and variety. A peanut butter and jelly sandwich can seem too easy to be healthy but it can be a great choice. Make a PB & J with whole grain bread, all natural peanut butter, and low sugar jelly. Try mixing it up by cutting the sandwich into interesting shapes or adding fun ingredients such as bananas or apple slices. If your child has a peanut allergy, you can use almond butter or any nut butter. Other healthy options are turkey wraps made with all natural turkey and whole wheat wraps. It does not have to cost you a lot of money to make your child lunches. In fact, it can be cheaper than buying them. Just prepare ahead.

Always include your child's favorite fruit, a healthy treat like a whole grain granola bar, and some flavored water. Try to stay away from pre-packaged and even portioned items. They might seem healthy because they offer fewer calories in a convenient package. However, many of these treats offer no nutritional value and a lot of sugar.

The best way to ensure that your child will eat that healthfully packed lunch is to get them involved. Give them some healthy options at the grocery store and let them decide what to pack for lunch. They want to feel that they decided what to eat. When you go grocery shopping, remember the kids' lunch. Have the food you want them to eat available.

KIDS IN SPORTS

Is there a safe limit of activity for children and teenagers? This topic is regularly discussed and argued by many physicians, trainers, and coaches. It is great if your child is physically active by means of a sports team or recreational activity. After all, a majority of our nation's children and teens are overweight. A study done by the Journal of American Medical Association found that 12.6 percent of thirteen-year-old boys and 10.8 percent of thirteen-year-old girls are overweight. In 2012 The National Health and Nutrition Examination Survey found that 18 percent of American children ages six to nineteen are overweight. And according to the government's Healthy People 2010, very few children are meeting the minimum daily activity requirement.

Roughly 40 percent of children have participated or are currently on a sports team. With the growing number of children playing sports and an earlier onset of sports training, it is important to find an appropriate amount of exercise and consider stress placed on the child.

There are many obvious reasons that exercise and sports related activities are good for a child. They decrease the risk of obesity and associated diseases including diabetes. Type 2 diabetes is commonly referred to as adult onset diabetes but more and more children are being diagnosed; a main cause is poor diet, lack of activity, high body weight/body fat. Exercise can also increase bone mineral density (BMD). The greatest amount of bone mineral density growth happens during puberty. The added stress of exercise combined with proper nutrition can increase a young person's bone density.

Weight-bearing activities such as running and jumping highly improve BMD and can help prevent the risk of future osteoporosis.

Regular exercise can also build the child's self esteem and confidence in their abilities. Playing on a sports team also teaches the child how to cooperate and work together as a team—a crucial lesson for success in all areas of life. Exercise can also improve mental focus and clarity in young children. It can provide a physical distraction from hardships and the stresses that are ever increasing in young children. Exercise can also increase insulin sensitivity in the body and help children sleep better. There are many other benefits to being physically active on a regular basis.

So what happens if your child's coach has them practicing every day and then they have a tournament all weekend long? Can your child overdo it and become injured?

An old belief was that too much stress on still forming epiphyseal growth plates would increase the risk of bone fractures and even stunt growth. This increased risk *is* present if the exercise is not supervised, performed improperly, or if the load is too great. For example, during weight training, teenagers must use lighter amounts of weight and stay in the repetition range of eight to fifteen. If a moderate level of intensity and frequency is used, then safety should follow. Just as with adults, children need time to recuperate and heal.

When excessive activity occurs, the body needs time to repair the damaged tissue or you end up in a vicious cycle of overuse. Overuse can lead to chronic fatigue and severe injury. Children could be more likely to sustain stress fractures and muscle sprains if proper warm-up and cool-downs are not performed.

The National Strength and Conditioning Association published a position statement in 2009 on children lifting weights and the proper time and implication for such an activity. They cite that resistance training can actually be a great form of exercise for those highly de-conditioned. Since weight training is not aerobic, then one can perform resistance exercise at a decreased intensity and still increase their muscular endurance and increase the fat free mass (muscle increase leading to a healthier body). They also document that children who participate in properly supervised and controlled programs come into their athletic sport more prepared and with a decrease in injury occurrence. NSCA recommends a child perform weight training two to three non-consecutive days of the week, performing one set of ten to fifteen reps as a beginner.

It is very important that you prepare your child for the physical, mental, and emotional stress they can endure during a practice or weekend tournament.

The three most important aspects to your child's preparation are sleep, nutrition, and physical readiness.

It might seem obvious that your child needs sleep. In fact, a typical ten-year-old needs ten to twelve hours of sleep per day! That might seem incredible but children are still growing. If they are highly active, they need quality sleep. If your child is involved in highly competitive athletics then it is imperative that they get rest. The body needs rest to ready itself for the next intense workout.

The best way to ensure that your child gets enough sleep is to stick to a bedtime ritual. As often as possible, stick to an early bedtime, even on the weekends. If your child misses a few hours of sleep each night during the week, then sleeping in one or two days on the weekend cannot possibly catch them up. Besides, if they have a completely different sleep schedule on the weekend then it is much harder to get them back on track come Monday. Most children typically do not get to sleep in. Therefore, a set bedtime is the best way to ensure proper rest.

Also, allow for downtime during the week. If your child is running around every day of the week and barely sits down until bedtime then you might be over-doing it. As a mother of two, I realize it is easy to have activities fill the calendar. Start saying no. Make sure that at least one night or afternoon a week is set aside for the children to relax. Plus, they will need some time to do their homework!

You also need to ensure that the child is receiving proper nutrition throughout the week for energy and muscle repair and regeneration. Children need at least 1,200 to 1,500 mg of calcium a day and a high dose of complex carbohydrates with lean proteins. Also make sure to feed your child large amounts of fruits and vegetables to increase their intake of fiber and essential vitamins and minerals.

It is ultimately the parents' responsibility to plan ahead. Sunday afternoons are a great time to prep for the week. Pack healthy lunches and after-school snacks that give your kids energy for sports practice. I suggest a snack with protein and complex carbohydrates. For example, peanut butter and an apple, string cheese and a banana, or a granola bar and chocolate milk. The great thing about low fat chocolate milk is that it offers protein, carbohydrates, and a little bit of fat and kids love the taste!

Hydration

Hydration takes days of replenishing and maintaining proper fluid balance in the body. It is extremely easy to become dehydrated. Losing just 2 percent of your bodyweight can cause negative side effects such as light-headedness, poor judgment, decreased motor skills, and slowed reaction time. Hydration is important for health and performance for all athletes but particularly for outdoor sports. To determine if you or your child is getting enough fluids to stay hydrated, you can perform the following sweat test:

- Weigh naked just prior to exercise, practice or game.
- Measure how much fluid is ingested throughout the exercise, practice or game.
- Immediately after, weigh naked again.
- For every pound lost, that is sixteen ounces (on top of what was consumed) that needs to be replenished. That means you should add sixteen ounces/per pound lost, on top of what was lost during the next practice, game, or exercise session.
- You will likely be unable to ingest enough fluid during exercise to prevent any dehydration, so make sure to replenish this entire amount of sweat water lost after completion of your exercise bout. You could weigh yourself each day. Weight lost within one exercise session is not fat loss; it is only water loss and should be replaced to prevent dehydration.

Research by the Gatorade Sports Science Institute shows that kids who are offered a flavored drink will drink more than if given just water. Try to avoid drinks high in sugar if your child is not active for more than an hour at a time. If the exercise session lasts longer than an hour, an electrolyte replacement is suggested. Try the new lower calorie sports drinks that still offer some carbohydrates, electrolytes, and water for rehydration.

Hydration should be a constant factor throughout the day. Make sure that your child carries water with them at all times. Check with your child's schoolteacher to make sure they can have access to water throughout the school day. It is very difficult to hydrate a child if they have been dehydrated for many hours. If they drink all of their water at once, they will be hyperhydrated. Most of the water will go to their kidneys and they have to use the bathroom instead of being properly hydrated.

Heat acclimatization

For those who have spent most of their summer days inside an air-conditioned facility or home, it can be very taxing on the body to jump into double practices out in the heat of the day. It takes roughly two weeks to acclimatize to heat conditions. Therefore, children who will be back on a sports field in the sun will need to get themselves accustomed to the heat slowly. Many schools have now adopted rules that prevent athletes from increasing time and intensity for long hours until they are accustomed to it. Teams generally increase time spent out in the sun each week throughout preseason.

Throughout the warmer months, you should heed the warnings signs of heat damage:

Heat exhaustion symptoms

- Pale with cool, moist skin
- Profuse sweating
- Muscle cramps or pains
- Faint or dizzy feeling
- Headache, weakness, thirst, and nausea
- Core (rectal) temperature elevated, usually more than 100 °F (37.7 °C) and the pulse rate increased

Heat stroke symptoms

- Unconsciousness or markedly abnormal mental status (dizziness, confusion, hallucinations, or coma)
- Flushed, hot, and dry skin (although it may be moist initially from previous sweating or from attempts to cool the person with water)
- Blood pressure may be high or low
- Hyperventilation
- Rectal (core) temperature of 105 °F (40.5 °C) or more

Muscle Conditioning

Proper activity level is set for children at sixty minutes, most, if not all days of the week. This type of activity does not have to be vigorous but something as simple as shooting hoops outside.

Depending on how much time it has been since your child played sports, it might be a good idea to start slowly. Remember that muscles grow and repair during recovery. So sleep and rest are just as important as the workouts themselves. Make sure your child eats a well-balanced diet and spends plenty of time resting and sleeping. This will allow their body to repair and be ready for increasing demands.

Even though most children are flexible, they still need to stretch, especially if their body has been pushed during the day. In the evenings when they are watching television or reading, remind them to stretch out (hold each stretch for about thirty seconds) to prevent some muscle soreness. Muscle soreness is normal and should not worsen after forty-eight hours. If pain persists days later and is confined to a joint rather than a muscle, you might want to see a physician to rule out injury.

Sports readiness

Make sure that your child is ready for the vigorous practices and schedules that the particular team or organization asks for. Many programs are highly competitive even when they are structured for young age groups. Just because your child is in that age group does not necessarily mean they are ready. Try to keep your kids active throughout the entire year so when a particular sport comes up, they are ready to participate. Find sports camps, after-school activities, or just get out there and play with them to allow them to enhance their skills before participating with a team.

Being the parent of a child athlete can be challenging. You are ultimately responsible for their health and wellbeing but you have to also think about their preferences. Enjoy their activities and remember that the healthier they are, the more fun they will have, the better they will perform, and the better they will feel!

Remind your children to advocate for themselves if needed. If they are feeling dizzy or faint during a heated practice, they should tell the coach. Every person comes into sports at a different conditioning level and will improve at varying rates. So make sure that your child knows that they should push themselves, but being cautious that their body might respond differently than a friend's body does. If you are uncomfortable with what is being asked of your child at practice, stay and watch to see what is really going on.

If you feel that the demands of a particular sports team or coach are too much, then remember that you can choose to have your child decrease their participation. It is a hard decision to make, but protecting their health is in their best interest.

EXERCISING WITH SMALL CHILDREN

Exercising regularly is very important to a mother's mental health and it can definitely make you feel better if you are getting your blood pumping. Yet if you have a baby, toddler, or small child, you know how hard it can be to fit in a workout.

When the weather is nice, it's a great idea to head outdoors for a few minutes of fresh air and exercise. If you have a jogging stroller, this can be a perfect way to relax the baby and burn some extra calories for mom. If not, then maybe your child is old enough that they can ride their bike while you jog.

There are some dangers with exercising outdoors. With some simple preparation and smart mechanics, you can prevent injury or harm. Exercising outdoors in the summer months with small children can present many hazards. First, the heat can be difficult for both the adult and child. Try to head out the door in the earlier morning hours or right before sunset when the heat index is lower and the radiant heat is less because the sun isn't at its fullest intensity. Usually before 10 a.m. or after 7 p.m. are good times, but in the height of summer, you might be safer off in the mornings as temperatures can still be very high in the evenings. Make sure to pack plenty of water for both mom and child. Even though your child might not be getting the calorie burn you are, they can get very thirsty. Wearing light colored clothing as well as sunscreen can help keep you cool and prevent sun damage.

There is always a risk from stray animals so I recommend carrying pepper spray and your cell phone. Exercise in a well-populated area and one that you could get quick help if needed. If a stray dog appears as you round a corner, take your jog down to a walk and don't run away. Dogs often judge your running away as a chase game. Instead, slowly walk to the other side of the street or path and calmly walk by. If you can calmly walk the other direction without spooking the dog, you can try that also. Your safety is more important than a preset route. It is also important to let someone know where you are headed and the estimated time of your return just in case. That way, they know where to look for you should something happen.

If you have a jogging stroller, there are many ways in which you can burn some calories and enjoy the outdoors with your child. It is extremely important to consider your walking and running form when pushing a stroller. It is very easy to slouch forward and round your lower back when you are pushing a stroller. Instead, focus on pulling your abdominals in and try to maintain your shoulders over your hips. Don't grip the handlebars too tight as this can cause you to slouch forward over the stroller. Maintain an upright posture as you push the stroller. If your child is heavier, and this is difficult, you can try pushing the stroller in front of you every couple strides. It is imperative that you use the safety strap around your wrist to prevent the stroller from getting away from you. Also, pull your chin down and back instead of projecting outward as this can cause neck pain and shoulder cramping.

Try these full body moves with the stroller at a park:

- Lunge forward uphill instead of running. This can be easier on your joints and build muscles in your legs.

- Park the stroller next to a bench and do some step-ups for some glute work.

- Sideways lunge with one hand on the stroller.

Last but not least, enjoy the time with your kids while getting healthy! You will look back and fondly remember these days!

KIDS AT THE GYM

With the childhood obesity epidemic on the rise, many parents are starting to encourage their children to increase physical activity. Naturally, since many of these parents belong to a health club, they invite their children to go along with them. But what are the health risks, if any, to young children participating in group exercise classes or exercising on gym equipment?

It is wonderful for parents to model healthy behavior such as physical activity and to invite their children to join them. There are several things to consider about kids being physically active. Does your health club allow young people to participate in the group exercise classes or to get on equipment? Some clubs have a minimum age for using exercise equipment and participating in classes. Often the minimum age to participate in a group exercise class is lower than that to get on equipment. This is due to the supervision of an exercise class that equipment might not offer. Group exercise classes can work for your child if you can supervise your child while participating and if you feel that various ability levels and rest breaks are allowed. High intensity boot camp and other militarist types of classes are too intense for many children.

If the class involves weight training, make an appointment with a teacher or trainer beforehand to see if there are any particular form issues to worry about. If there are many people in a class, and the instructor is stuck up on stage, help with form might not happen and your child risks a serious injury. Ensure that your child uses a very light weight. It is commonly recommended that children not use external sources of resistance (bars, dumbbells) until they are in their teens. Prior to that, weight training should be just with bodyweight resistance. Cardiovascular activity classes can often be safer for children if rest breaks are incorporated and various levels of activity given.

Yoga can be a good fit for children due to the slower nature of the movement and more controlled environment.

The maturity of your child will also play a large role in the risks that might be encountered. If your child seems to be mature and act responsibly, they might perform better in a health club setting then a child who has problems listening to rules and obeying property with respect and knowledge. Children using cardiovascular or weight training equipment can often be dangerous if the child is not properly supervised or trained on how to use it. Parents need to stay with their child at all times in a weight room and supervise all activity. If you are not comfortable teaching your child good form, hire a trainer to get them on a program that is appropriate for their age and ability.

Again, young children should not be using heavy, external resistance for risk of damaging growth plates or soft tissue. The weight room can be a very dangerous thing for some children and many gyms have age limits that deter young children from the area. If your child is a teenager, then they can begin to learn proper form and use lighter weight when working out.

Make sure your child is properly dressed for activity. They need to have comfortable shoes and breathable clothing as children sweat less and have more difficulty regulating body temperature. Have your child drink plenty of fluids before, during, and after exercise to maintain hydration. And couple exercise with healthy nutrition. Give your child plenty of recovery if a class or workout was strenuous.

If the exercise activity starts to get boring to the child, then change it up. Let them pick what they get to do and make sure they enjoy it. You do not want to create an aversion to physical activity at an early age. Physical activity should be fun and there are many things a child can participate in at the gym and outside as well!

SUMMER FITNESS

The history of summer vacation from school used to include many forms of physical activities. It used to be that summer meant children riding bikes, swimming, and out shooting hoops until the sun went down. Now, children often lack a safe place or the motivation to get outdoors and get moving. Instead, children are often sitting indoors, watching television or surfing the internet on their computers.

When kids are in school, although they are usually sitting, they are often away from food and take part in some form of physical activity such as recess or physical education. When at home during the summer, kids are not instructed to be as physically active and they have easy access to food. Kids often gain fat weight in the summer months and lose physical strength and stamina. However, children in outdoor camps and organized programs are often able to maintain or even increase physical activity.

If you can afford it and have transportation for your children, it is a great option to sign your kids up for a sports camp or outdoor camp. Usually, city recreation departments, local health clubs, boys and girls clubs, and universities offer camps.

If camp is not an option, there are still several ways to help your child stay active. The first suggestion is to limit screen time with your children. Children ages two or over should not watch more than sixty minutes of television a day. Total screen time of television and computer or video games should not equal more than two hours. Let your child pick one or two of their favorite shows or games and limit screen time to their chosen show. Next, give your child possible replacement options that involve physical activity.

Children can do many activities indoors if safety outdoors is a concern. You can purchase inexpensive items for young children such as hooks hoops, jump ropes, and balls to play with. For older children you can purchase an exercise video and have them do it a few times a week. There are many exercise videos for sale online, which vary in type and intensity. Make sure your teenager or child helps you pick it out so you know they will use it.

You can also take turns with other parents to supervise children playing outdoors at a park or local field. If one parent can take a group of children once a week, then it might feel more feasible to get them outdoors daily.

Children can also be assigned various household chores that will keep them moving and help you around the house. This is another area largely missing from many children's summer activities. Kids can learn how to help the family unit and gain responsibility. Getting the kids to take part in the weekly vacuuming, sweeping, dusting, and window cleaning can get them moving and decrease the time you have to spend cleaning instead of being with them. Provide a sticker chart of chores that they can complete during the day. If, at the end of the week, they have filled the sticker chart, then you can reward them with a trip to their favorite park, maybe the zoo, or another fun outdoor activity (just don't make the reward food oriented!).

Swimming in a safe environment is also a great form of activity for children in the summer months. Make sure that the area is safe and it is best if your child has a high level of swimming ability if no life guard is present. Try to avoid any moving water for leisure swimming as this can be dangerous to children. Swim lessons can be a great life skill for children and provide for them wonderful activity.

CHAPTER 10

AGING

You are never too old to exercise. In fact, more and more research points to the fact that exercise can help slow down the aging process of both your mind and your body. Studies have shown that a decline in physical performance and lean body mass is associated more with a loss of activity than it is associated with aging alone. The USDA's Agricultural Research Service recently reported on the elderly and their improvement with exercise.

The USDA cites a study done at Tufts University in Boston, in conjunction with the USDA Human Nutrition Research on Aging, which was performed on 213 people aged seventy to eighty-nine years old. At the beginning of the study all subjects were sedentary. They found that after a year, those who exercised 150 minutes or more per week had the most improvement.

Another study done by the USDA Human Nutrition Research on Aging found that subjects that were given at home exercise programs improved in cardiovascular endurance and walking speed. And these participants who showed improvement were also sedentary and not participating in physical activity prior to the study protocol. Their research protocol lasted only six months and there was significant improvement in balance, which is very important for the aging population.

Balance is vital to the elderly population because 9,500 deaths occur each year in older Americans due to falling. Thirty percent of hospital admissions of the elderly are due to falling. In fact, persons sixty years and older have a 30 percent chance of being hospitalized due to falling and persons eighty years and older have a 50 percent chance of hospitalization due to falling (for those who live independently). Falling can often lead to breaking a hip or other osteoporotic bone areas and this can lead to being bedridden. Hospitalization and lack of mobility can lead to more serious complications such as pneumonia and sometimes infection. What is even worse is that once a person has been hospitalized, the chances of being hospitalized again increase. Once a person has been hospitalized from a fall the chance of falling again is one in five for the older populations.

Exercises that improve balance and stability are vital for overall health and independent living for the older population.

Another very important reason to exercise is to increase strength. Increasing body muscle mass and strength decreases the risk and severity of osteoporosis and can improve core strength, therefore leading to a lesser risk of falling. If you do have osteoporosis, then it is advised that you utilize a clinical specialist in this area to get specific exercises that work around your complications and risks. Spinal twisting of any kind is not recommended for those with osteoporosis.

Research by Peterson, published in Medicine and Science in Sports found that older women can improve their strength just as much as younger women can. They tested a group of women who were eighteen to thirty-three years old and another group of women who were sixty-four to eighty-five years old. Both groups performed the same resistance exercises. After eight weeks of training, they found that the older group improved their strength just as much as the younger women did. They did not see as drastic an improvement in muscle power, however that could be somewhat due to muscle fiber size and neuromuscular firing. Therefore, people of all ages can improve their strength.

If you are new to exercise, it is highly recommended that you get a physician's clearance first. Then find a qualified professional trainer who is skilled in the area of older population training and understands the various differences in this age group. You could ask your physician if they recommend anyone or shop around for what feels comfortable. If you have severe osteoporosis or osteoarthritis, then you should consider exercising in the pool to get your body acclimated to exercise again. If you want to try resistance training, work with a certified professional. I suggest starting with just one or two nonconsecutive days a week of training and perform only one set of eight to ten reps with very light weight. You want to learn proper form first!

The best thing you can do for your heart and overall health is to get out and walk. If your balance is not good then find a track with a handrail for balance and be careful if you walk outdoors. Make sure you take someone with you in case of an emergency. There is no exact number of minutes you should walk. Just do what you can and take breaks when you need to. Also, sip water throughout exercise to prevent dehydration. And finally, find a friend who wants to exercise with you. Make it fun and explore different types of activity with your partner. You might be surprised how enjoyable exercise can be at any age.

RUNNING IN LATER YEARS

Do you think it's too late to start really exercising? Are you thinking, "I'm too old to start something like jogging now?" Or, "jogging or vigorous activity could cause me harm like bad knees or injury?" These are many myths surrounding aging and exercise.

Many researchers have focused decades on studying the effects of exercise on the aging body—even in your eighties and nineties! Henriette van Praag in the journal Trends of Neuroscience, 2009, published findings that exercise increases blood flow to the brain and could even reduce the likelihood of dementia and Alzheimer's disease. Physical activity also decreases depression and anxiety amongst the older population.

Surprisingly, researchers have shown that running can actually decrease your risk of knee pain. In 2008, a study was published in the American Journal of Preventative Medicine that showed that those who ran did not higher prevalence of osteoarthritis. They followed over 100 people ages fifty to seventy-two years, half runners, half not runners (control group) from 1984 to 2002. It is hypothesized that knee pain is associated with aging because of loss of muscle strength, power, and flexibility. With aging often comes a more sedentary lifestyle and this causes a loss of muscle fibers. This in turn can cause problems such as knee pain, back pain, and difficulty doing activities of daily living. In fact, researchers at Tufts University found that patients who already had diagnosed osteoarthritis felt a 46 percent decrease in pain as a result of regular physical activity (including weight training) for sixteen weeks.

When it comes to the benefits of regular exercise, researchers in Germany found that strength (resistance) training, two to three times per week, has positive effects on risk factors for cardiovascular disorders, cancer, diabetes, and osteoporosis. In September 2005, in the Archives of Physical and Medical Rehabilitation, Kingsley reported that elderly female patients who performed strength training for twelve weeks reduced fibromyalgia pain and had an increase in strength. Alfieri in 2010 published a study in Clinical Interventions of Aging that when patients who were older than seventy-years-old were trained in postural and strength training, they saw a marked decrease in falls. This is very important because people over sixty-five years old risk falling at least once a year without an intervention. Researchers believe that lifting weights at 65-75 percent of your maximal voluntary weight is sufficient for increasing strength and bone mineral density.

Before Beginning:

Check with your doctor first if you:

- have a cold, flu, or infection accompanied by fever
- have significantly more fatigue than usual

- have a swollen or painful muscle or joint

- have any new or undiagnosed symptom

- have chest pain, or irregular, rapid, or fluttery heartbeat

- have shortness of breath

- have a hernia, with symptoms

- have been advised by your doctor not to exert yourself for a given period of time due to illness, surgery, etc.

How to Get Started If You Feel Past Your Prime:

- Start with using light dumbbells doing things like squatting into a chair and back up, pressing the weights over your head, and getting up and down off of the floor. These are all things that help you increase strength for everyday activities.

- Try to do two sets of ten repetitions for your exercises. If you can do more than ten repetitions, you should lift heavier weights.

- If you cannot do at least eight repetitions, then lower the weight of your dumbbells. It is important to lift heavy enough weights to create an overload on your body but you want to make sure to keep good form.

- Count two seconds as you lift or exert and four seconds as you lower to ensure good form.

- Stay consistent. We all get busy with vacation or illness, but get right back to exercising as soon as possible.
- Lift weights two or three non-consecutive days of the week to give your body ample rest time.
- On the days in between, you can go for a walk.

MAINTAINING STRENGTH IN LATER YEARS

It can feel like it is much harder to make gains in muscle strength and tone as you increase in age. While it is true that it can become more difficult to maintain muscle mass and overall figure as you age, there are things you can do. Although many people worry about the loss of muscle mass that affects their appearance, there are many other risks to losing muscle mass. In 2006, Robert Wolfe, American Journal of Clinical Nutrition, reported that loss of muscle mass can increase your risk for osteoporosis, mortality, and morbidity (disease and loss of quality of life).

During the years of puberty, the body starts to rapidly increase the production and release of natural anabolic (building up) hormones. Hormones such as testosterone, estrogen, elastin, collagen, and human growth hormone all play key roles in puberty. When puberty hits and these hormones are increased in circulation, the body starts to put on more muscle mass and exhibit secondary sex characteristics. As a person goes through the lifespan, such hormones will decrease in production and in secretion. Therefore, the body has a harder time building up muscle tissue and tends to show signs of aging. Also, years of free radical damage from sun exposure, possibly alcohol or tobacco products, and other unnatural additives, your body will show more signs of aging such as wrinkles, loss of skin elasticity, and subcutaneous fat. Skin often becomes thinner and the body will more easily pack on pounds of fat tissue (due from decrease in hormone levels). But what can you do to help prevent muscle tissue loss and improve your fitness and physique? There are many things you can do and some possible supplements that have been argued to help.

Current researchers have argued that increasing muscle mass during the latter years of life can decrease morbidity and improve quality of life. As well, a loss of muscle mass will increase your risk for diseases such as osteoporosis which is a weakening of the bone tissue. If you are smaller framed and lose muscle mass then your risk for osteoporosis increases as well as your risk for bone fractures of the hip and back.

Regular weight training can help you maintain and possibly improve your muscle mass. Everyone should aim to do at least two to three days of moderate to intense resistance training. Once you have received clearance from your physician, it is wise to have a full body routine that you can realistically complete at least a couple times a week. The moves should incorporate your whole body.

Stay away from the easy to use machines if possible. Every time you sit to do an exercise, you are using less muscle to perform the task. Try performing as many activities as you can on your feet and using your entire body. Get a trainer to help you if you are not sure about proper form. The old fashioned basics are still great moves. Try push-ups, lunges, and pull-ups. If you are using weights, make sure you are using a weight that is heavy enough to fatigue you at twelve repetitions. If you can keep going much past this, you might not be stimulating the muscle enough to elicit a response. Since older bodies need more recovery time, make sure to spread out your weight training days by at least forty-eight hours. If you don't think you are pushing yourself hard enough during each workout, hire a trainer to show you the intensity at which you need to work.

Nutrition is another key to a healthy body and this can become even more important as you age. You might feel like your metabolism has slowed; this can be due to a loss of muscle. Eat a high amount of lean protein, complex and natural carbohydrates, and healthy fats such as flaxseed and olive oils.

Some claim that supplements such as DHEA can help increase muscle mass and the appearance of older skin. The National Library of Science states that your body can produce DHEA and that it does not need to be taken through supplementation unless your doctor has prescribed it for the treatment of lupus or osteoporosis.

Necessary supplements could include calcium, vitamin D, and amino acids. They might be able to improve your overall nutritive intake.

PREVENTING FALLS

Falling is the most common reason for hospitalization of older populations. It is extremely common for people to fall more and break bones as they age. This is due to several factors including bone mineral density, balance, and lack of strength. What can you do to prevent this from happening to you? There are many things you could do in and out of the gym to help prevent the chances you will fall or that you will break a bone.

As we age, we have a loss of balance and strength. Balance can be challenged through various exercises. If you tend to lift weights sitting on machines, learn to do more resistance exercises standing up or on a physioball or balance disks. When you sit to do all of your resistance exercises, you are not training your core and stabilization muscles like you would if you stand or sit on an unbalanced surface. So try doing lunges with your feet on balance discs, perform overhead shoulder press while seated on a ball, and even try standing one-legged to perform some upper body exercises. To really push your balance, try taking small hops up and down on one foot to train your proprioceptors (muscle receptors) within your foot and leg.

Decrease in strength can predispose you to falling. One of the greatest muscles that decrease in strength as we age is the gluteus medius muscle and other muscles that help abduct your leg (move your leg away from your body). When your leg does not properly abduct with each step during your gait, you increase your risk for falling. These muscles reduce in strength because we don't often perform abduction or lateral movements as we get older. We tend to do our daily tasks in a straight path that does not require much lateral movement and we sit often which can weaken our gluteals and tighten our adductors (inner thigh muscles).

To strengthen your abduction muscles, do lateral squats. Starting with feet together, step to the right into a squat and repeat four times. Then return back in the other direction four times. If this is too simple, place an elastic band around your knees while you do this to increase the resistance and therefore increase the strengthening potential of your abductors. To increase the strength of your gluteal muscles, perform step-ups onto a bench with a height about an inch below your knee.

If you lose muscle strength then you have a higher risk of losing bone mineral density. Weight training—along with adequate nutrition—can help prevent bone mineral density loss. Make sure your calcium intake is close to 1,000 mg of calcium a day (it's best to spread it out in two or three doses of 300-500 mg each). By performing weight training, your muscles put strain on your bone and therefore cause more bone growth to occur. This will help increase your bone mineral density. Without doing resistive exercise, you will most likely lose a large amount of muscle strength and lean mass after your twenties! It is necessary you place demand on your skeletal system to keep your bones strong.

If you are already working out regularly, I suggest you incorporate balance exercises at least once a week, resistance training at least two times a week, and ensure you are getting enough calcium along with magnesium and vitamin D. Bone loss, called osteoporosis, can also run in the family. If your parents had smaller frames then you could also have a smaller frame. If you tend to be petite and smaller, your bones could also be smaller, and more prone to osteoporosis. Have your bone mineral density checked if you are unsure about your risk.

CHAPTER 11

HEALTH FADS

We live in an age when everyone is wanting the quickest and easiest way to a better body and health. We all want an edge; an advantage over others to achieve peak performance or quicker fat loss. There are numerous fads, some beneficial and some not. It can be very difficult to determine fad from fact and the best way to determine if something is myth and fad is to unearth the best evidence based facts. It should take more than one author, or one study, to change a basic gold standard practice. You should be able to see multiple authors and articles in agreement when you are choosing to start a new diet, exercise program, or nutritional supplement. Insure that the risks do not outweigh the benefits when researching a new health fad.

HIGH ALTITUDE EXERCISE

High altitude exposure can provide many positive benefits to cardiovascular and respiratory performance. After exposure to higher altitudes, exercise at sea level will often feel easier and you will fatigue later. To explain why, you first must understand the differences at high altitude.

As you travel up in altitude, atmospheric pressure drops, air has lower density, and there is a reduced partial pressure of oxygen. That means that at sea level with atmospheric pressure equal to 760 mmHg with 20.6 percent oxygen, there is 159 mmHg of oxygen (PO_2 = 0.2093 x 760 mmHg = 159 mmHg). At an elevation of 9840 ft., total barometric pressure drops to 526 mmHg and therefore the partial pressure of oxygen is 110 mmHg. When the partial pressure of oxygen drops, the ease at which your lungs fill with oxygen lowers. Normally, at sea level, your lungs easily fill up with air because the partial pressure of oxygen in the atmosphere is higher than it is in your lungs and gases naturally move from a place of higher concentration to lower concentration. At higher altitudes, the partial pressure of oxygen is lower and therefore does not as easily diffuse into the lungs as it does at sea level. The percentage of oxygen at high altitude is the same, but the pressure of it decreases due to atmospheric pressure decreasing.

Researchers have found that 10,000 feet (or 3,048 meters) is considered high enough to elicit a physiological response to altitude. During one bout of exercise at high altitude, only acute (immediate) responses will be felt. Examples of acute responses are hyperventilation, increased viscosity of blood, and increase in heart rate. Chronic (longer-term) responses can occur if a person trains at high altitude for at least two weeks for 2,300 meters—with an additional week for every increase in 610 meters. Chronic adaptations are decreased submaximal heart rate, increased blood plasma, increased myoglobin (to carry oxygen to muscles), and increased mitochondria (part of cell that helps produce energy).

Some scientists and exercise physiologists suggest the "live high, train low" program. This means that an athlete should train at lower elevations and simply live at higher elevations to elicit the same positive physiological response. The reason is that if an athlete only trains at higher altitudes they could begin to muscle waste, begin eating away at iron stores (decreasing myoglobin/hemoglobin), and become dehydrated.

For the average person hoping to improve their general fitness, it might not be worth it to travel to a higher altitude to train. You might see a slight change in physiological response but much of it could be due to an increase in physical activity, not altitude. Try training hard for a race or event at whatever level you live at or plan to compete at. That is probably enough to gain the benefits you want. If you are looking for an edge over other competitors who might live or train at higher altitudes, you could try altitude training, but remember it takes at least a couple weeks to elicit a long-term response.

ANTI-INFLAMMATION DIETS

We often associate inflammation with swollen ankles or the stiffness of arthritis. For example, in rheumatoid arthritis, the body responds with inflammation and the immune system attacks the joints. While these are examples of inflammation, there are other, more recently discovered causes and symptoms of inflammation in our bodies. Inflammation is often a chemical and structural reaction in our body to foreign or dangerous substances. The foreign substance can be bacteria, stress, or diet related. Recently, inflammation has been researched for its affects on heart disease, obesity, and disease risk.

Cardiovascular disease risk is one of the most common areas of inflammation research. Researchers found that an inflammation marker, called C-reactive protein, is elevated in people who have heart disease. When artery plaque causes a clot formation, the response to this clot is inflammation. This inflammation causes blood levels of C-reactive protein, and has become a marker for arthrosclerosis and coronary events.

In a study called "Monitoring Trends and Determinants in Cardiovascular Disease," 1,000 men ages forty-five to sixty-four were followed for eight years. The study found high levels of C-reactive protein were associated with coronary artery disease. A study at Harvard Medical School found that drugs, like pravastatin, could lower C-reactive protein levels. More common drugs to decrease inflammation are non-steroidal anti-inflammatory drugs (NSAIDS) such as Advil and Ibuprofen.

If you want to lower your coronary artery disease risk without drugs, you can try an anti-inflammatory diet. What is an anti-inflammatory diet? It consists of eating certain foods that lower and lessen inflammation in your body. The absolutely worst thing to eat for controlling inflammation is processed food. High-sugar and high-trans-fat foods actually increase your body's inflammatory response. In an anti-inflammatory diet, omit processed, high-sugar foods. Research shows that you should also stay away from foods with high levels of a chemical alkaloid called solanine. Solanine is found in some vegetables like potatoes, tomatoes, and eggplant. Too much red meat can also trigger inflammation.

However, many vegetables and fruits are the best thing to decrease inflammation. To decrease inflammation, increase your intake of Omega-3 fatty acids. These are found in walnuts, flaxseeds, canola oil, olive oil, and cold-water fish such as salmon. Also increase your intake of berries, particularly strawberries and blueberries, which have high levels of antioxidants. Soy products such as soymilk and tofu have shown to reduce inflammation, as do high fiber foods. Get your high fiber foods from whole grains such as oatmeal or 100 percent whole-wheat products. Increasing green-leafy vegetables might decrease inflammation. Drinking herbal tea can also be anti-inflammatory. Be sure to drink a lot of water to combat inflammation.

Exercise can also help reduce inflammation by improving healthy cholesterol (HDL) and improving circulation. The combination of exercise and a diet of anti-inflammatory foods and without processed foods, should help decrease your body's inflammation.

Exotic Fruits

Many companies tout the benefits of ingesting exotic fruits such as acai and goji berry. Acai berry is native to the Amazon rainforest, looks like a small grape, with a taste that some say is a mixture of blueberry and chocolate. Acai berries are high in polyunsaturated fats, dietary fiber, Vitamin E, calcium, potassium, magnesium, and anthocyanins (antioxidants found in the dark purple, grape color). The acai berry itself deteriorates rapidly so it is often found dried or in smoothies. Goji berry, also known as wolfberry, is a bright red-orange fruit found in China. It is rich in fiber, riboflavin, copper, iron, potassium, and zinc. This berry is high in beta-carotene, lycopene, and zeaxanthin (all antioxidants).

Antioxidants help fight free radicals that can often cause cell deterioration and the signs of aging such as wrinkles. If you want to slow the effects of aging and increase cell regeneration then you should increase your intake of antioxidants. The big question is: are antioxidants in acai and goji berry better than more traditional berries such as blueberries? A study published in the Federation of American Society for Experimental Biology in 2007 discussed the antioxidant level in subjects after acai berry pulp ingestion versus an antioxidant juice mixture. Those subjects who ingested the acai berry pulp had up to 50 percent higher levels of antioxidants in their blood plasma.

The USDA tested over 100 foods for their antioxidant capacity and found that berries in general won for the highest antioxidant capacity. Wild blueberries were the winner with 13,427 antioxidants in one cup, which is ten times the USDA's daily antioxidant recommendation. Next on the list were cultivated blueberries with 9,019, cranberries at 8,983, and blackberries at 7,701. Strawberries, plums, and even Granny Smith apples recorded high levels of antioxidants. Sifting through the research, the jury is still out on whether acai berry is really higher in total antioxidants and its absorption in comparison to other berries. In fact, a study performed at

Texas A & M found that acai berry pulp was absorbed at higher concentrations in subjects than applesauce, so acia berries high antioxidant levels can be used by the body. It is very questionable if the difference in cost is worth the small increase in benefits. It all depends on how much money you have and how hard acai berry juice is to find. You also have to check if the juice is 100 percent acai.

Goji berries have also been touted to have the same antioxidant benefits. The claim is that goji berries stop DNA cell damage and decrease the risk of certain diseases. Some research shows that goji berries improve brain function and health. Goji berries have eighteen amino acids, unsaturated fats, and zeaxanthin, which is a carotenoid that is contained in the retina of the eye. However, if you take blood thinners such as Warfarin or if you take diabetes or blood pressure medication, then you might not want to eat too much goji berry, as some studies show a negative drug interaction.

The benefits of these two berries are said to be high and effective ranging from decreasing risk for cancers, aiding in weight loss, and even decreasing risk of Alzheimer's. The question is how reliable and valid these studies are when performed by those who have vested interest in the berries' consumption. Many antioxidant foods can benefit your body.

BLOOD TYPE DIETS

A book titled *Eat Right 4 Your Type* by Dr. Peter D'Adamo, a naturopathic physician, has sparked a buzz on whether various blood types require and reject certain types of foods. The idea is that your blood type—A, B, O, or AB—helps determine appropriate foods for you to eat. Foods are then categorized as super beneficial, beneficial, neutral, allowed frequently, and avoid. D'Adamo has a website that allows you to easily explore the claims of such a diet (www.dadamo.com). In D'Adamo's defense, his website is chalked full of research articles that aim to prove his theory. Yet the research conclusions vary and many of the studies cited are his own. Therefore, he could have some warranted theories, more research by non-involved parties would be beneficial. D'Adamo says that "blood groups can provide insight into seemingly unrelated aspects of physiology, including variations in intestinal alkaline phosphatase activity, propensities toward blood clotting, reliability of some tumor markers, the composition of breast milk, and several generalized aspects of the immune function" (2001). The main focus is on lectins, proteins that are on the surface of foods that cause molecules to stick together. It is argued that these lectins adhere to your muscle tissue changing acidity and deteriorating muscle function. Evidence such as muscle biopsy would help the reader feel more convinced that such a drastic event could happen if say you ate too many legumes and were Type O, as the book claims.

Many participants of this program would persuade you that it is the best diet they have gone on, improving immune function, weight loss, energy, overall health, and even curing of ailments. However, the Mayo Clinic even reports that this diet has no foundational basis and might not provide enough nutrients.

There are other books such as one written by Joseph Christian called, *Blood Types, Body Types, and You* that follow the same basic premise. However you still need to look at the facts before diving in. Some red flags of these types of diets were found in a review of D'Adamo's book, *Cancer: Fight It With the Blood Type Diet*. Registered dietitian, Alen Mierzejewski, reviewed the book and uncovered that there are no conclusive research data included in the explanation for using such a diet.

If you are a blood type diet believer, please remember that oftentimes fad diets work. You could try this diet and feel better, have more energy, and experience a healthier life. However, this could be simply because you are now conscious and aware of what you are eating. This diet does emphasize eating mostly healthy, natural foods for all blood types and that can help improve your health. It is common nutritional knowledge that what you eat does highly effect how you feel. You will feel much more energetic eating naturally raised foods compared to processed and manufactured foods.

If a diet such as this helps you start to eat healthy foods and cause you to become proactive in your health then that is great news. Make sure you are getting a well-balanced diet full of healthy fats, lean proteins, and complex carbohydrates that vary in color.

Finally, make sure that a nutritional program you start is one that you could continue for the rest of your life. If you are still unsure, ask your physician. They are usually your best resource and can help you determine if a particular diet or lifestyle is best for your medical history and current situation.

DIET PILLS

The greatest way to weight loss that lasts is adequate physical activity and healthy nutritional intake. Unfortunately, there is no quick fix to weight loss. The weight loss products sold in the supermarket are not always the best answer to weight loss and can even possibly harm your body. However, this is not preventing Americans from buying supplements to help their venture toward health. In 2009, Americans spent $33.9 billion on supplements.

Weight loss products sold in the drugstore are not tested or regulated closely by the FDA like prescription medications are. That means that a diet pill is not tested for its safety or efficacy. One of the only ways these items are regulated is through their labeling capabilities. Nutritional supplements, including diet pills, are not allowed to claim that they treat or cure any diseases. However, their labeling can make similar claims such as "helps lessen symptoms" or "may promote weight loss...." If a product claims to help you lose substantial weight in a short period of time then it is probably too good to be true.

Back in the 1970s, popular stimulants phentermine and ephedra were marketed to the public for obesity treatment as Fen-Phen. In 1996, a New England Journal of Medicine article cited a twenty-three-fold increase in hypertension (pressure in the pulmonary system) when a person was on Fen-Phen. One maker of ephedra containing products, Metabolife, received 14,000 complaints of adverse effects. Cases of heart problems, and even deaths were reported, causing a stop in the sale of Fen-Phen in 2004. Ephedra's herbal name is ma huang. Ma huang is a traditional herbal stimulant used to treat things like hay fever, but was found to increase heart rate and help with weight loss. Therefore, ephedra started to be included in diet pills due to its ability to increase metabolism. The United States has very loose control of dietary supplements (diet pills and other supplements) and therefore, this herbal stimulant was not tested prior to its being sold by the millions in the U.S. market. The FDA has very little control over the production and sale of dietary supplements due to the Dietary Supplement Health and Education Act of 1994, which does not require testing of dietary supplements including anything that is intended to supplement the diet. Therefore, just because something on the shelf does not have ephedra in it, does not mean that the ingredients were scrutinized in a laboratory prior to its sale.

So what ingredients do diet pills contain now? Common ingredients in diet pills now are caffeine, taurine, tea extracts, and other herbal supplements such as Rhodiola rosea extract. Roots such as rhodiola can often be used for increased energy and alertness. There is less research and longitudinal data on newer traditional roots and herbal extracts being used as diet pills, and the verdict is still out. Some studies have shown adverse effects with ephedra free supplements such as Xenadrine EFX. The American Journal of Medicine found a 7 to 12 percent increase in blood pressure with the use of ephedra free diet pills.

Many diet pills contain caffeine, guarana and/or ma haung. These products are all stimulants that increase your heart rate and can lessen your hunger. This might cause short-term weight loss but the risks are high. Too many stimulants racing through your system can cause heart palpitations and chest pains. The drug ephedrine has been banned from supplements because of its link to heart attacks. The other stimulants used in diet pills are not necessarily safe just because they are not banned.

Many diet pills contain stimulants that also act as diuretics. This causes you to lose a lot of water weight. So most of the weight that you might lose in the first few weeks would not be fat weight but water weight.

The way many diet pills work is that they mimic your body's natural hormones epinephrine and norepinephrine. These are your fight or flight hormones that cause your heart rate and blood pressure to naturally increase to cause a surge of energy in case of the need for survival. One theory is that when you have stimulants like ma haung or guarana in your system for too long, your body will start to lessen its natural production and release of its own hormones epinephrine and norepinephrine. So when someone stops taking diet pills, their body is still not producing enough of its own hormones and they gain weight. Again, this is just a theory but it points to why people often gain weight after they stop taking diet pills. Many diet pills caution customers to only use the pills for a short time. Your body will become dependent to the stimulant effects and you can end up going through withdrawal type effects if you take them too long.

For some people the effects may not be noticed but are still harmful. When your blood pressure is elevated from an herbal supplement this means that arteries are constricting from a pharmaceutical agent, not physical exertion. Increased blood pressure is a signal of constricted arteries and this increase in systemic pressure (pressure in the arteries), means that the heart has to work harder to push against that resistance to get blood to the entire body. When the heart is forced to push harder, there is a chance for harm to the heart. As well, long-term increases in blood pressure can be harmful to your cardiovascular system.

The conclusion is that diet pills are not the best answer to long-term weight loss. It is better to stick to a well-developed exercise plan for the rest of your life. That does not mean you have to kill yourself at the gym every day. It means that fitness and health is a life-long journey and you should look at activity as a part of life. If you take diet pills and do not change the core root of your weight loss struggles then you will not lose weight and keep it off. You need to deal with the things that cause you to fall off track and lose focus of your goals—even if you take a supplement. If all you do is take a diet pill, then you risk not losing weight or not keeping it off. Try to incorporate fitness into your life in a realistic way that enables you to lose weight and keep it off.

If you have any lingering question as to what the long-term effects of diet pill use is, try using the old-school method of weight loss: eat less, move more! It is not easy and not always the quickest way, but it is advised as the safest way to lose weight.

CREATINE

Creatine monohydrate supplements are used to help enhance the ability to increase strength and muscle size. Creatine phosphate is used in the body to produce energy (ATP) for short burst activities such as lifting weights or a short sprint and therefore, creatine supplementation is thought to work on this system by feeding it more creatine, and therefore, more energy. Creatine monohydrate increases the muscles' retention of water and often causes the user to notice their muscles being fuller or "pumped" which explains the immediate pay-off visually. However, the increase in water retention could possibly cause compartment syndrome and with habitual use, kidney damage.

Football and baseball athletes are the highest users of use such supplements. However, no organization has recommended the use of creatine for anyone under the age of eighteen. In 2010, a group of McMinnville, Oregon, athletes were hospitalized with what is called compartment syndrome.

Exertional compartment syndrome is the result of swelling of the muscle tissue within the muscle sheath, or compartment, of an arm or leg. If pressures rise too high, nerves and muscles within the compartment may be permanently damaged. If there is concern that the pressures are potentially dangerous, the compartment can be opened to relieve the pressure and avoid nerve injury. It was found that the athletes were taking supplements of creatine but a direct link between creatine use and these hospitalizing syndromes was not made.

A study published in the Journal of Athletic Training in 2006 studied the effects of creatine monohydrate supplementation and the association with compartment syndrome. A group of athletes were given twenty grams/day for seven to ten days, a typical loading cycle, and measured for compartment syndrome. It was found that those who exercised in the heat, and were therefore more dehydrated, had higher risks of compartment syndrome. Body water is taken up by the muscle cells and increases the risk of dehydration and possibly, compartment syndrome.

Young people who are still growing are at increased risk of harmful side effects of supplements and should not ingest them without the recommendation and approval from their physician. Although creatine supplementation might not cause compartment syndrome or other side effects, it could contribute to the likelihood of an unwanted physical effect. Young persons should focus on obtaining overall fitness, and strength within the confines of a safe and functional program, supervised by a professional coach or trainer.

YOGA

Yoga has been around for thousands of years and yet recently it has received a lot of attention because of the star appeal. Many Hollywood stars are telling the media that they obtain their svelte figures through healthy eating and devotion to practicing yoga.

How can yoga be better than sweating like crazy for hours on the treadmill? The answer to that question lies in the total body effect of yoga, not the amount of calories burned in the single workout. On average, an hour of hatha yoga burns roughly 130 to 220 calories an hour, depending on your weight and intensity. An hour of ashtanga or Bikram yoga can burn more in the range of 250 to 400 calories an hour. To compare, if you run on the treadmill for thirty minutes at 6.0 mph, then you will burn roughly 350 calories. Ashtanga and Bikram yoga are more intense practices of yoga that involve quicker succession of poses and muscle toning moves. Bikram yoga is done in an extremely hot room, which intensifies the workout.

There are many benefits outside of the sheer calories burned during your yoga session. Persistent yoga sessions, no matter what the form, are extremely beneficial to your overall health. Researcher Satyajit R Jayasinghe published an article in 2004 in the European Journal of Cardiovascular Prevention and Rehabilitation supporting the effects of yoga on cardiovascular health. Hatha yoga not only improves flexibility but also can strengthen the heart and increase immune function in post-myocardial infarction patients (heart attack patients).

A study performed by the American Council on Exercise (ACE) showed that women who practice fifty-five minutes of Hatha yoga three times a week increased their flexibility by 13 percent and increased muscular fitness.

Can yoga lead to weight loss? The American College of Sports Medicine (ACSM) stated in their news release in 2003 that yoga sessions could lead to weight loss. They cite that weight loss requires a calorie deficit so the intensity at which you practice yoga is important. Another important factor in weight loss through yoga is the relaxation effects. When we take time to focus on deep breathing, meditation, and relaxation, then we are more likely to make healthy eating choices. When we are stressed we often reach for unhealthy comfort foods. So when you take the time to practice yoga you then meld the mind with the body. You allow your mind to slow and that in turn allows your heart rate to slow and your digestion system to work more effectively. When you are more content and relaxed you will not misinterpret being stressed for being hungry.

Use yoga as a part of your fitness routine. Try to perform five to ten different yoga poses three times a week. Try the sun salutation series and deep breathing techniques and hold each pose for fifteen to thirty seconds. Give yourself a peaceful and quiet place to perform this routine. If you are new to yoga, then try receiving one-on-one help from a certified yoga instructor or take a class from a reputable instructor. You want to make sure that your yoga instructor has been trained by a certified licensing trainer in the specialty they are teaching. The more hours and experience your yoga instructor has, the more comfortable you should feel with the quality of training you are receiving. There are many different forms of yoga training so make sure that your instructor has gone through a program that not only requires instruction but also observed hours by the certifying agent. The instructor should have logged hundreds of hours of observed instructing before leaving the program.

Instead of opting only for the treadmill or only for the yoga mat, do both. Your mind and body will like it!

FITNESS TECHNOLOGY

In our busy lives, it can be difficult to track workouts, determine progress, and find new ideas for working out. It is often said that technology has made us lazier over the years. Remote controls allow us to change the channels without getting up; email allows us to converse with a coworker without leaving our cubicle; and drive-through restaurants give us food with no effort. But technology has now begun to afford us luxuries that can help us meet our fitness goals! With the invention of smart phones, notebooks, and iPads, we now have apps for anything, including fitness and exercise!

There are pros and cons to using technological apps for fitness motivation. The benefits include specific workouts, a mobile tracking ability, and minimal boredom since many of the apps have a large variety of tools. One of the biggest benefits of many mobile apps is that they also sync with an account you can open on any desktop computer, making it easy to see your progress, share it with others, and even print things like running routes.

Some of the possible disadvantages of an app are that they are still a computer, not a real person. A real person will have great success at getting you up and working to your full potential when a computerized gadget might be easier to switch off or put away! You will most likely feel greater guilt when blowing off your personal trainer or a friend in a group exercise class, than you do turning the reminder off of your latest fitness app.

If you are looking into buying a fancy gadget such as a GPS tracking watch, you should consider its pros and cons as well. The benefit is that many GPS tracking watches also have heart rate monitor capabilities and can sync to a computer. This is a great feature for goal setting and training. However, you should really be sure you plan to use that GPS watch often and for a while as they can be very pricey (i.e. Garmin Forerunner starts at $399)! Another GPS gadget is the Nike GPS chip that can go in a shoe and track where you have been and the pace you have been at. Nike has a few different watch options with GPS. Some of their basic models at $100-200. This is very user friendly and easy to use since you don't need to carry anything cumbersome with you!

Which apps are worth your time and storage space? Here is a great breakdown of the best fitness related apps and the best ways to use them.

- **Basic fitness and weight management:** MyFitnessPal (free). This is a great app that also syncs with an account you can look up online. It customizes how many calories you should eat and burn through exercise each day to reach your weight goal. It gives you many activities to choose from and then credits you those calories burned for the day (available on iPhone and Android).

- **Workouts with limited equipment:** Boot Camp Challenge ($3.99 iTunes). This app has over 200 exercises to show you based on the equipment you have on hand. If you only have dumbbells it will give you a workout that includes only dumbbells as the equipment necessary! It shows you exercises in video format so you can be sure to nail perfect form.

- **Yoga-enthusiasts:** Pocket Yoga ($4.99 iTunes). This is great tool with more than 140 poses you can pick and choose from to create your ideal yoga routine.

- **Intense workout routine:** P90X for iPhone ($59.99 for entire package or about $6.99 for one group). This app shows you videos of all of the P90X exercises but it will cost you for each series. There is also a crossfit app called Pocket WOD that will give you daily workouts and it's free!

- **Runners/Cyclists:** MapMyRun/MapMyRide (free). This is an amazing app that allows you to use it as a GPS tracking device, logging your workout, distance, and pace as you go or you can create a mapped routine from your desktop computer. You can use this app on iPhone, Android, iPad, and your desktop. Each one syncs to the same log-in and allows you to see progress from anywhere. This app also lets you tell friends on Facebook or Twitter about your latest run or share routes with people all over the world.

- **Healthy/Wholesome eaters:** Intelli-Diet App ($3.99 iTunes). By telling this app what you have in your kitchen or what your preferences are, it will create an eating menu and grocery list from wholesome, natural foods that will help you meet your weight loss goals.

Tips for choosing your best app:

- What is your favorite activity? This will help you determine if you want a GPS tracking device for jogs or a weight lifting app.

- What is realistic for you? If the app requires minute-by-minute logging, you might quickly forget or get overwhelmed by it, leaving you frustrated and not using the app at all.

- If the app costs money, will you keep that mobile device for very long? Will it transfer to another device if you upgrade soon? If you have both an iPhone and iPad, some apps only work on the iPhone and not the iPad, so look closely before downloading.

- Ask around to see what others like or dislike. Some apps can be very user friendly and others not. So ask your friends and family what they like and see if they think it is worth the money.

CHAPTER 12

HEALTH INFORMATION SOURCES

INTERNET HEALTH INFORMATION

N ow more than ever before, you can hop on the internet and answer any health or fitness questions you have. Most of us have questions regarding why our knee hurts when we run, how to cure a headache, or how many calories we should eat in a day. But can you get valid information just by typing your query into a search engine? The unfortunate thing is that practically anyone can post practically anything on the internet and therefore there is way too much information that is not worth reading.

Information is valid if it actually answers the asked question appropriately. Many websites are simply one person's opinions and are not grounded in scientific truth. So how do you know the difference? Check for Credibility, Accuracy, Reasonableness, and Support (CARS).

There are a few ways to determine if an internet site contains valuable or invaluable information. The first and most basic thing to look for is the author. Who wrote the article and what are their credentials? Are they certified or licensed by a nationally or internationally acclaimed organization? What experience and degrees do they have? Of course, people can have credentials and yet know very little about the topic or they can impose opinion and not fact into their writing.

Now look to see if the information has references listed. Adequate references should be listed at the bottom of the article or page and the references should be from peer-reviewed research journals, not magazines. Peer-reviewed journals are those in which each published article is read and critiqued by many experts; only valid and reliable research is published. Magazines are not high quality evidence for any health guidelines. The best websites provide an exact link to each reference so you can read the entire article from which the information comes.

The website should list when it was created and the last date it was updated. Contact information for the author should also be listed.

Good information is also collaborated and supported by other organizations or review boards. Look for gold standards in care. Examples would be ACSM (American College of Sports Medicine) for exercise, AHA (American Heart Association) for cardiac problems and rehabilitation, NATA (National Athletic Trainers Association) for athletes, and AAP

(American Academy of Pediatrics) for children's issues. If you go directly to these sources, you will find the latest and most accurate information.

For general information I recommend these websites:

- www.webmd.com for WebMD – the most comprehensive information regarding various health issues.

- www.cochrane.org for the Cochrane collaboration – a global effort to summarize the best and latest information regarding health.

- www.pubmed.gov – this website leans to the more clinical side of health but can offer some information on specific injuries, illnesses, and treatments.

These websites are just a few to go along with the other gold standard organizations mentioned above. If you can, always go to the direct source of information. Search for peer-reviewed articles that have been published in a reputable journal and not in a popular culture magazine. Remember that anyone can write a blog online but you want to look for a reputable author who has been published in a journal.. If you are not sure where the website information came from, you need to find the source or else disregard the information.

Remember, while some magazines can offer some valuable tips and tools, they are not the primary source of information. They should not be considered the final say in any major health issue. If you are researching to self-diagnose, you might end up more injured, confused, and frustrated. If you are not sure, go see your physician. The internet is a great tool for information but should not be taken as fact. Dig deep to determine the source and make sure the source has gone through a rigorous analysis!

TELEVISION HEALTH INFORMATION

Similar to the internet, reality shows are not always reality. For example, *The Biggest Loser* is a show where extremely overweight contestants compete to win a large cash prize. The show is centered on weekly weigh-ins, challenges, and voting off a contestant. There are many positive things about *The Biggest Loser*. The show is making a huge impact in educating people about the importance of exercise and healthy eating. It emphasizes the need for conscious awareness of what we eat and how little we move. While the show provides some great exercise motivation, it might not be the best in exercise reality. For example, is losing twenty pounds in one week possible or healthy? Yes, some contestants have done it on the show, primarily in the beginning weeks of the contest. But are you capable of results such as this at home? Probably not, and I would not recommend it.

One of the most unrealistic parts of the show is the amount of time the contestants spend exercising each day. In reality, no one has that much time to exercise. Only the contestants on the show who are living at the Biggest Loser camp, far away from their families, jobs, and friends have time for this. Their daily exercise is their full-time job. The rest of us have full-time jobs and kids to chase after so we are lucky to get in thirty to sixty minutes a day. So you probably can't burn the amount of calories they burn.

Some of the contestants went from doing absolutely nothing physical to exercising eight hours a day—their bodies are bound to drop some serious weight! For some people, after losing a large amount of weight in a short period of time, they hit a wall and stop losing so quickly. Losing a large amount of weight in just a few days can be attributed to water weight loss and also can be hard on your body.

Research shows that the quicker you lose weight, the more likely it is that you will gain it back. Our bodies do not do well with large weight loss. If you restrict your calories and lose a lot of weight you might also slow your metabolism down and that will eventually backfire. You might have heard the trainers on the show say that the contestants are not eating enough. For the contestants, they are used to eating upwards of 6,000 calories a day (before the show). Then they start eating fewer calories of much more nutritious foods and lose a lot of weight. Their bodies are going through severe change. If you cut your calories to lose and exercise too hard, then your body will revolt and quit losing weight. Your brain will assume you are working your body to death, burning a lot of calories and not eating enough, so it will store what you do eat as fat. The lesson for us is to reduce calories enough to lose about one to two pounds a week, not the twenty that you see on the show. Eat a diet full of natural and nutrient rich foods and eat every few hours to keep your metabolism working efficiently.

When it comes to exercise, you need to try to be active everyday: as little as thirty minutes or as much as one and a half hours. Some of the exercises that the contestants perform on the show might not be safe for everyone. I do not suggest anyone riding a leg press machine for weight as I have seen on the show. This is not safe and not allowed in most gyms. I also think that high impact exercise such as jumping and running might not be worth the potential knee damage if you are considerably overweight. If you are quite overweight, focus on low-impact exercise such as swimming and walking until you lose some weight. This will lessen your joint pain and ensure that you can continue exercising for the rest of your life, not just a few weeks of insanity.

Remember that we live in reality, not on any TV show. Set up your diet and exercise program as one that is balanced and adequate to perform for the rest of your life!

PERSONAL TRAINERS

If you can afford the time and money, a personal trainer is your best bet for guidance for a workout program. Certified personal trainers have specialized skill sets and experience to provide you safe and effective programs. If you do not want to pay for a gym membership and a personal trainer, explore the possibility of using an at-home trainer who can work with you in your home on your schedule. When the New Year rolls around, you might also be able to find some special deals on personal training packages.

Hiring a personal trainer can be a big decision. It is a time and financial investment and one that should be thought through. If you feel like you have reached a plateau or slump in your workout routine, or if you getting over a major injury or rehabilitation program, working with a personal trainer might be the only way to get a safe and effective workout.

The benefits of a personal trainer are lengthy. One of the biggest benefits of hiring a personal trainer is the structure of each workout. Workouts can get tedious and boring and often inefficient if they are left to you wandering around the same weight room. We are creatures of habit and we often do the same exercises whether they are proving to be effective or not. We like to feel safe and comfortable with what we are doing and that often means our minds and bodies become bored with the monotony of the workout! A trainer can guide you through a variety of exercises with the knowledge to teach you proper form.

The next benefit of hiring a personal trainer is the opportunity to learn the correct form for all prescribed exercises. I cannot tell you how many times I have seen people perform exercises in faulty and often dangerous bodily movements. It is incredibly important to learn the proper way to execute an exercise. For many of us, it is not enough to simply watch someone do the exercise and try to mimic it. We often miss some very important details that could provide a more effective and safe way of doing it.

One of the greatest benefits of a trainer is often perceived as a deterrent: trainers cost money. If we are investing money into time with a trainer then we are more likely to show up for our workouts. After all, they are waiting and we are paying for it! This is helpful for many people who struggle to get to the gym consistently. Of course, this is not enough of a reason to pay the money if you are not seeing results after a while, but it can get you in the habit of exercising regularly.

If you have a particular physical goal (rehabilitation from a surgery, finishing a triathlon, picking up your grandkids after a back injury), then a qualified personal trainer could help get you there.

If you decide that hiring a personal trainer is an investment you want to make, then there are some things you should look for beyond big biceps.

Things to look for in a personal trainer:

- Look for a trainer who **walks the walk.** You don't want a trainer telling you to cut out junk food while they eat potato chips in their office. If they aren't living a healthy lifestyle, they will not have much empathy or understanding for you.

- The **basic qualifications**. A degree in exercise science or a related field is very important, as is a certification through a nationally recognized certifying organization like ACSM, NASM, and NSCA. A great trainer is continuously being educated on the latest techniques. Ask the potential trainer what their last workshop or training was and what they learned.

- **Relevance.** Ask the trainer to describe a past client who had similar goals to you and how they turned out. Find out about their successes and failures and how they would change things. This will show you the trainer's strengths and weaknesses but also give you an idea whether or not they are willing to continually improve their specialty.

- **Personality and training style.** Watch a trainer at your local gym with their current clients. Are they attentive to the individual's safety, goals, and style? Some trainers are yellers; others are quiet encouragers and you will want to know what type of trainer matches your desire to be pushed. You can usually tell by watching a trainer if they are the type of personality you would want to pay for!

- **No strings attached.** Find out if you can do a couple of trial sessions before signing on for a long commitment. You don't need to feel badly about this. Once you choose a trainer, give them all you have since your only results will come if you are fully committed. But if you find that your personalities are not a good fit or they are not the quality of trainer you expected, then you should have the option to find someone else.

- **Be straight forward.** This is for your safety and health! Ask them what they know about any physical conditions or injuries you have had. Do they have a good rapport or partnership with a reputable physical therapist?

You shouldn't judge a book completely by its cover. I did say you should find someone who walks the walk but just because a trainer looks good doesn't always mean they know how to train you or have much knowledge of the body or nutrition. Ask for references and see if you could possibly talk to any of their current clients to get an idea of their experience.

No matter what, hiring a trainer for either the short or long term will help you reach your goals safely and effectively. If money is an issue, then hire someone for a small amount of time to get yourself going. A trainer could be a great investment in your health.

CHAPTER 13

EXERCISE GADGETS

Technology has infiltrated the health and fitness world and it is every changing. Therefore, by the time this book has gone to print there will inevitably be a slew of new gadgets that I have not included. I hope to have included some of the more pertinent and well-established gadgets that you will find useful and affordable. Do some research on any new gadget before purchasing it? Determine if there is a return policy, ask what reputable health professionals say about the gadget and how long you will be able to use it. Many gadgets like Suzanne Somer's Thigh Master was popular but was ineffective and had a very short shelf-life. If something costs a lot of money, then be certain that you can utilize the gadget for a long time!

MYOFASCIAL RELEASE

There is a lot of talk and hype about massage sticks, balls, and contraptions. Giant foam rolls, lacrosse sized balls, and massage sticks are found in all athletic facilities such as physical therapy clinics and health club gyms. All of these tools have the same common goal: muscle fascia release.

Fascia is a structure of connective tissue that surrounds muscles, groups of muscles, blood vessels, and nerves. The function of muscle fascia is to reduce friction to minimize the reduction of muscular force. Fascia provides a sliding and gliding environment for muscles, suspends organs in their proper place, transmits movement from muscles to bones, and provides a supportive and movable wrapping for nerves and blood vessels as they pass through and between muscles.

Myofascial release is the massage and release of the fascia that surrounds the muscles and often impedes and restricts normal movement and range of motion. Often times, you can use tools or hands (often knuckles) to apply pressure to trigger points or areas where the fascia is tight to help release the tightness over time. Myofascial release and massage can be performed either by a clinician or by yourself.

We develop tight fascia through everyday repetitive movements and exercise. Over time, our fascia becomes more and more taunt and it can be impossible to stretch it fully with manual self-stretching as we would our muscles. If we do not release the fascial tension, then we could likely end up have restricted movement and compensate elsewhere in the body, often leading to injury. Fascia often gets tight and restricts movement in areas such as the lower back, hips, and shoulders.

Everyone could benefit from doing myofascial release techniques but if you have persistent tightness, pain, or shortened range of motion then you could be in serious need of this technique.

Physical therapists and licensed massage therapists can massage the tissue and therefore release adhesive restriction that can occur with tight fascia. Another way to perform myofascial release is through self-massage using either a foam roller, ball, or massage stick. Before trying any of these tools, remember the following tips from Michael Stanborough, author of *Direct Release Myofascial Technique: An Illustrated Guide for Practitioners*:

- Land on the surface of the body with the appropriate "tool" (knuckles, forearm, etc.).
- Sink into the soft tissue.
- Contact the first barrier/restricted layer.
- Put in a "line of tension."
- Engage the fascia by taking up the slack in the tissue.
- Finally, move or drag the fascia across the surface while staying in touch with the underlying layers.
- Exit gracefully.

Key myofascia release tools

- Foam Roller: comes in a variety of densities (high density, low density, grid, and EVA foam for heavy use).

- Massage Sticks

- Lacrosse balls: these are great for digging into trigger points.

More recently, trainers are teaching clients to do trigger point therapy with a grid roller. A grid roller is designed to hold heavy individuals. It has zones that mimic the human hand and has sections to simulate the palm and finger-like area of a massage therapist. These zones give a deeper massage, to allow oxygenated blood flow to the tissues. Grid rollers especially aid aging athletes in circulation and flexibility. You can buy a grid roller through online distributors such as Amazon.

The best time for you to perform myofascial release and massage is prior to your exercise routine, as part of your warm-up. This helps lessen the tensile resistance of the fascia and allows for a freer range of motion during your activity. If you can, perform full body foam and ball rolling out as shown in the photos. Move slowly through a large range of motion.

Foam rolling technique

When using a grid roller, focus on the areas that you know are tight and restricted. Begin at the top of your body and move down. The more body weight you rest on the foam roller, the more intense the pressure will be. If you are supporting your body with your arms, you will want to maintain good spinal alignment (don't let your back be kinked to one side or the other).

Self-Massage Techniques

- IT band roll out: Place outside thigh on top of the foam roller and slowly roll the leg up and down, extending up past the hip and down beyond the knee, to work into the tight fascia that lines the outside of the thigh.

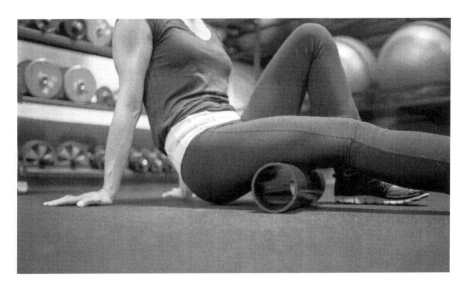

- Calves and hamstring roll out: Roll the entire back of the leg back and forth along the foam roller.

- Massage stick lower leg: Push and glide the massage stick up and down the lower leg, along the front muscle along the shin and up and down the outside of the calf to release the tired muscles we use in walking and jogging.

- Glutes and piriformis: If you have tight glutes and any sciatica, this could help you. Place the lacrosse ball under your glutes until you find the "sweet spot," where you feel tension deep under the gluteal muscles. Lie flat and continue deep breathing to release.

- Neck and tension massage: Put the lacrosse ball against a wall and then lean back into the ball. Let the ball find the tight knots and spots along your shoulder blades and lower neck (trapezius muscle) area.

ELASTIC BANDS

Have you ever used the excuse that you don't do resistance training because you don't have the money for a health club membership? Or that you can't spend the money on an at-home weights set? What about the excuse that you travel a lot so you don't have constant access to weights? Well, make no more excuses.

Did you know that resistance training is crucial for maintaining and improving total body lean muscle mass and bone mineral density (decreasing osteoporosis risk), increasing your metabolism, and getting the toned body you want? The American College of Sports Medicine recommends that you get at least two non-consecutive days of resistance training, with eight to ten different total body exercises. However, it can be difficult to fit in resistance training when you are also trying to do that recommended three to five days a week of cardiovascular exercise. Some people shy away from resistance training since it requires some instruction and equipment. Health club weight rooms can seem intimidating and prevent you from getting in there and trying anything. And if you are not a gym member, then you have to learn how to get a good workout in at home.

Elastic bands are a great at-home exercise tool that will help you incorporate a full body resistance training routine that is inexpensive and effective. Elastic resistance tubing was first introduced as a physical therapy modality and has since been modified for use in all types of exercise moves. Elastic allows for increased resistance and effectiveness for your workout.

Elastic tubing will give you resistance throughout the range of motion you are performing.

Although elastic tubing without handles has been the standard in therapy clinics, if you are purchasing tubing for the following exercises, it is recommended that you purchase tubing with handles.

How to shop for tubing: color and size

Bands are not described in pounds but in tension. Most companies have five or more different tension intensities ranging from very light to extra heavy. Each company offers color-coded bands to match the degree of tension. A general rule is the lighter the color, the less tension (i.e. yellow is often very light and dark blue is often extremely heavy). You might need more than one tension as you will likely need higher tension for your lower body and lighter tension for your upper body. You can also manipulate the tension of a band by changing the placement of your feet. Anchoring the band with one foot lengthens the band, which allows it to "feel" lighter than placing both feet on the band to anchor it.

Complete the following exercises with your tubing, at least two non-consecutive days of the week. Complete a five to ten minute warm-up prior to beginning the routine. If you have a past injury, get physician approval prior to starting this program.

It is very important that you have secure placement of the band before beginning to prevent injury.

Exercises:

- Squat with a row: holding the handles of the bands in each hand, arms straight with resistance on the bands, slowly squat down so thighs are parallel to the floor. Once in the squat position, then row your arms by bending your elbows and pulling them back while squeezing your shoulder blades together.

- Lunge with overhead press: Stand in a lunge position, one foot in front and one foot behind with the center of the band underneath the foot in the front and the handles of the band in each hand. Lunge down so the front knee bends to 90 degrees while you press your arms holding the band up and over your head.

- One-legged chest flies: Wrap the band around a fixed and stable surface at chest height. Face away from the object holding the band with band in each hand. Balance on one foot and perform chest flies with the band, bringing your hands together in front of your chest at chest height and then draw them out away from you. Repeat.

- Side lateral raises: Stand on the center of the band. With each hand holding an end of the band and elbows slightly bent, bring your entire arm up and parallel to the floor so that wrist, elbow and shoulder are at the same height. Slowly lower and repeat.

- Bicep curls: Stand on the center of the band, hands holding the ends with palms facing forward, curl your hands up to your shoulder while keeping elbows stationary by your side performing a bicep curl.

- Triceps extension: Standing on one end of the band and holding the other end in one hand, extend arm straight over your head with your arm next to your head. Keep your upper arm next to your head while you slowly lower your forearm and hand down and back bending your elbow. Make sure to keep your elbow up by your head. Then straighten your arm to return your hand straight up.

FITNESS STRAPS

Most people want an exercise program that includes serious muscle sculpting moves without a lot of equipment and a gym membership. Besides elastic bands, one of the greatest inventions is the fitness strap, the trademarked commercial name is TRX straps, which allows you to use your own body weight for major muscle sculpting. These straps are gaining popularity by all workout enthusiasts.

Fitness straps use what is called suspension training that incorporates your entire body. Since you are using your own body weight and you can adjust the straps to fit your intensity level, almost anyone can utilize these straps to produce a wonderful resistance-training program. You can perform resistance training, cardiovascular exercise, core, and stabilization moves to enhance all areas of your body. They are often seen in health clubs but if you buy a pair you can easily do the following moves on your own at home with the help of a sturdy place to affix them.

If you are new to fitness straps, purchase a beginners or home-starter kit. Starter kits often include DVDs or a beginner's guide that will teach you the basic moves, and all of the essential parts to starting correctly. You can even purchase a mount for the straps if you do not have a strong place to put these in your home.

The Best Exercises:
- **Heel to Butt Stretch:** Lying face down on a bench, one leg extended behind you and the other bent so that hip is flexed and foot is on the ground underneath you. Place a strap around your extended foot. Gently straighten and bend the extended leg pressing your hips into the bench to increase the stretch in the quadriceps and hip. Do 5 repetitions and switch legs.

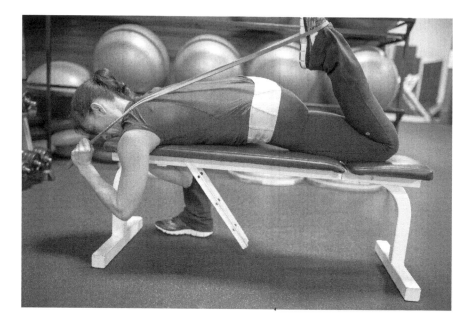

- **The Pendulum:** To get your abdominal muscles firing, put your feet in the straps and your hands in a push up position. Keeping your abdominals in and your back flat, gently swing your legs from side to side to activate your obliques and all core muscles. Complete as many repetitions as possible.

- **Single Leg Squat:** Facing the straps and holding one in each hand, stand on one foot. Then slowly sit back into a one-legged squat and gently rise to standing. Repeat ten on each leg. Make sure you drop your hips back and keep your knees tracking in line with your toes.

- **Pull-ups:** With a strap in each hand and facing upward, put your body in a plank position just off the floor. While maintaining a flat back, pull your body up in a rowing motion while elbows are drawn back. Slowly lower your body. Repeat ten times.

- **Push-ups and flies:** Face down toward the ground with your back flat, weight resting on your toes, and a strap in each hand, then push your body up and down as done in a push-up exercise. If you can succeed at this exercise for ten repetitions, try chest flies by extending your arms out to each side, as you would do in a dumbbell fly exercise. Repeat ten times.

- **Mountain Climbers:** Place a foot in each strap and your hands in a push up position. Keep your abdominals in and back flat, then jog your feet in and out for ten seconds and progress up to thirty seconds.

- **Hip Extension Hold:** Lay on your back with your heels in each strap. Keep your body aligned while pressing your hips up toward the sky. Hold for ten to thirty seconds.

Get approval from your physician before you start a program with fitness straps. If you have had back injuries, definitely seek physician approval and increase the intensity very slowly. Strap workouts are wonderful for a full body workout but do rely heavily on your core (abdominals, back, and hips) so you want to warm up prior and make sure you have ruled out any injury restrictions.

Fitbits/activity watches

Activity monitors in the form of wrist worn watches and bands has become extremely popular. There are Fitbits, Nike fuelbands, and other activity watches on the market. Many of them only track your activity like a pedometer, counting your total steps taken and miles walked in a day. This can be a great way to see if you are meeting the recommendation of 10,000 steps, roughly 5 miles, a day. However, the only way to track your intensity of activity is to wear an accelerometer that will track the speed at which you are moving throughout the day and even during a planned exercise bout like a run. Both are valuable tools for tracking personal physical activity however which one you will find most helpful will largely depend on what you are trying to track. If you are interested in seeing if you are getting vigorous activity over low intensity exercise you will need something that works more like an accelerometer and not just a pedometer.

Many of them will sync with a desktop program or software that can increase the way in which you can compare your daily activity or even compare with others. I have used

Nike Fuelbands and Fitbits and have found benefit in both. A
Fitbit is easy to wear since it is small and is easy to charge. As
well it easily syncs with software on a desktop for tracking
daily activities and sleeping patterns. The Nike Fuelband gives
you access to a large database of thousands of other people
tracking their activity. It can be fun and inspiring to log onto the
Nike Fuel site and see your progress along with many others.

CHAPTER 14

BUDGETING FOR HEALTH

I t can be extremely difficult to see the value in spending a limited amount of income on something that seems as "selfish" as a gym membership or physical therapy. However, spending a relatively small amount of money now could save you thousands of dollars in medication and healthcare bills later.

It is estimated that the average American in 2014 spent more than $8,000 a year on medical expenses. Americans spend more than two and half times what other developed nations spend out of pocket for personal healthcare expenses. This is coupled with higher rates of heart disease and obesity than many other nations. (It should also be said that America's health system is making big strides in improving infant mortality rates and improving the quality of life for chronic diseases such as some cancers and heart disease.)

The International Health, Racquet, and Sportsclub Association (IHRSA) reports that 44 percent of gym club members quit their membership because of the cost. As well,

58 percent of people who are not gym club members state that they do not join due to the high cost. US News reports that the average monthly gym membership is $55. That is an average of $660 per year. Many diet programs such as Weight Watchers cost around $42.95 for an in-person membership or $18.95 for online support. This can quickly add up to quite a bit of money. But let's go back and compare that to the $8,000/year an average American might spend on health care!

A large percentage of the medical costs in America are due to modifiable conditions such as obesity and type 2 diabetes. In the United States alone, we spend $245 billion on treating diabetes. These costs are from inpatient care, prescription medications, physician office visits, and diabetes supplies. The Centers for Disease Control and Prevention (CDC) reports that people with diabetes have medical costs two and a half times greater than those who do not suffer from diabetes. Type 2 diabetes can largely be controlled and prevented with weight management, exercise, and appropriate nutrient intake. Therefore, putting money into your health could actually save you financially in the end.

Another factor to consider is missed workdays due to illness. Regular moderate exercise can improve your immune function, which can therefore reduce the risk of you getting sick and missing work. For many people, that means a higher income.

Regular exercise can also boost your mood and give you mental clarity. This can improve your quality of life and your productivity. If a gym membership is something that is truly a luxury in your budget, then you should still consider getting out for a daily walk. And if you can put a few more dollars toward healthy foods instead of convenience foods, you will reap the benefits.

Living a healthy lifestyle will help teach the next generation—especially your children or grandchildren—to do the same, which is good for the whole community.

EATING WELL ON A BUDGET

Sometimes it can feel challenging enough to get any kind of food on the table, let alone a meal that is healthy. Although healthy food has a reputation of being expensive, you can easily buy foods that will be good for your family's health without breaking the bank.

It's essential to think about the health of your family through the foods that you buy and prepare. Why is it important? Childhood obesity is on the rise. In 2014, the CDC reported that 21 percent of kids twelve to nineteen years of age and 18 percent of kids ages six to twelve were obese. Obese means that the body mass index (a ratio of height and weight) is over the 95th percentile. Childhood obesity can predispose an individual to type 2 diabetes, high blood pressure, high cholesterol, heart disease, osteoarthritis, and even asthma. If you want to prevent your child from joining this large percentage of our childhood population, then your efforts are well worth the extra resources.

With a grocery store full of options, what are you to do with it all? The best recommendations are to first shop the perimeters of the store, staying away from the aisles that harbor processed foods. Second, I suggest checking out the bulk food sections where many items are to be had for much less money than in a box.

At the perimeter of a grocery store lie the produce, meat, and dairy departments. You can obviously make poor choices in the meat and dairy departments but there are also many healthy items there as well. In the produce department, try to buy at least three to five fruits and three to five vegetables. Be brave in trying new things such as sweet potatoes, beets, and turnips. All root vegetables can be chopped and roasted in a 400-degree oven to create a simple but tasty way to eat vegetables. Also stock up on a couple of leafy greens such as broccoli, kale, and salad greens (preferably not iceberg lettuce).

If your children go with you to the store, let them pick a new vegetable to try at home. If they are part of the shopping and choosing process then they will be more likely to eat the vegetables once they are prepared. If you aren't sure about a produce item, seek out the produce department manager. They can easily tell what various options are and even how to prepare them.

You can always get your usual bananas and apples but try being adventurous in the fruit department as well. Has your child tried kiwi, fresh pineapple, or fresh peaches? Most of the time you can get an enormous amount of fresh produce for a fraction of the cost of canned fruits or vegetables. You will be saving money and your family will be getting a healthier dose of vitamin-rich produce. Canned items are usually full of either sodium or sugary syrup so fresh is much better and even cheaper.

In the meat department, look for whole roasting chickens or large meat portions such as pork loins. You can buy a lot more meat for the same amount of money if you buy it in a large portion rather than always buying chicken breast or cut pork loins. You can roast a chicken in the oven for meat that can last your family a few days.

In the dairy department, you can often buy light yogurt for the same price as regular and skim milk for the same price as 2 percent. Check with your pediatrician, but most children can switch to 2 percent milk after their second birthday or sooner. Also look for low-fat and low-calorie options for sour cream, cream cheese, and coffee creamer. If you are looking to save some money, buy your cheese in a block and shred it yourself.

The bulk section is my favorite area. You can often find inexpensive and organic versions of oats, roasted (but not salted) nuts, cereals, and whole-wheat flour. Buying food in the bulk section will save you a fortune off of what the manufacturers want for the same thing in a pretty box.

Finally, plan ahead. Go to the store with a list and a plan for the week ahead. Stick to your healthy list and avoid processed foods that just look tempting. Get one or two treat items such as non-fat pudding and low-fat ice cream sandwiches for those special times. And eat before going grocery shopping. If you are hungry you will end up filling your cart with numerous things you were not intending to buy!

BUDGETING FOR A GYM MEMBERSHIP

In a down economy, wallets are pinched tighter and tighter and people cut back on their spending. And one of the first things to cut back is your gym membership. That is especially true if you see it as a luxury item or you rarely use your membership. There is logical thinking about getting rid of any unnecessary bills during a time of economic hardship. Perhaps a gym membership feels like something you could once afford and now cannot. Or perhaps it was once something you valued and it isn't a value to you anymore. Before you cancel your membership, ask yourself: what is the value of this membership to me? Do I use the membership now? Will I miss it and have to pay a cancellation fee as well as a new join-up fee if I decide to go back?

The cost of terminating a contract can be over $250 and if you later decide to rejoin, you could face another $100-$200 joining fee. Those put together are a lot more money than possibly hanging on to your membership.

Outside of looking at objective data such as dollar amounts, let's look at the benefits to a gym membership. A gym membership allows you to put your money where your mouth is. If you value health and want to get or stay in shape, than your money is well worth being spent on a membership. Your health often requires an investment. Just paying the membership does not help you get in shape. It is actually going to the gym and burning off those calories that helps you get in shape!

You can also look into a health savings account with your employer. Many companies now offer these types of accounts that let you file claims for preventative healthcare and might help pay the bill of your gym membership. That would use tax-free money that you have set aside every month to pay for items such as these. Check with your employer.

One of the biggest benefits of having a gym membership is the community and camaraderie. It is very difficult for most people to exercise at home alone. It can be very difficult to motivate yourself and get the exercise and intensity you need on your own. A gym often has a multitude of exercise classes that can motivate you as well as teach you new ways to work out. If you are a beginning or infrequent exerciser, then you probably need that motivational factor in the gym and group atmosphere. Having others around you can help push you to work harder than if you were alone in the garage.

The other issue is just getting on your exercise clothes and doing it. When you have a set time to get to the gym to meet with a trainer, start a group exercise class, or meet up with a friend, you are much more likely to follow through with it. Without that appointment, you are on your own and more likely to talk yourself out of it. So keeping your gym membership can be beneficial if you lack self-motivation. If you are highly motivated and have a workout partner for outside the gym then you might do okay.

If you weigh out the pros and cons of keeping or quitting your gym membership, you should be able to make a decision you feel good about. If you decide to forego the membership, then I suggest you prepare in order to not fall into bad habits. Create a workout plan that will work realistically in your life. That means scheduling exercise on your calendar like you would time to go to the gym. It needs to be written in your day timer, put on your outlook, or set on your smart phone. Whatever you have to do to make it a priority in your busy life, do it!

Have the proper tools to be successful. Find a partner who also wants to work out on his or her own time. Schedule at least two of the five workouts a week with that partner to keep you accountable. You can even do weekly weigh-ins with each other to stay accountable! Next, get the equipment you might need. If it is as simple as buying new walking shoes and clothes, then do that. Often times new workout clothes will motivate you to wear them and get moving. If you want to exercise in your home by yourself then purchase an exercise ball, some weights or resistance bands, and maybe even an exercise machine like a bike or treadmill. If you believe you are going to stick with an exercise program at home then the investment might be worth it. If you cannot stand the thought of exercising on a machine alone then you might think about putting your machine in front of the television. That way you can pass the time faster. Buy some exercise videos to help guide you through a workout program or tune into the television channel Fit TV. This channel gives you 24 hours of exercise shows ranging from yoga to cardio and weights.

EPILOGUE

Phew. Take a deep breath. There is so much information here: so many ways in which we can get active, maintain a healthy body weight, and better our health. Do not let the massive amounts of information become paralyzing and overwhelming. Take baby steps. Small, yet consistent steps toward a healthier you is what will make a difference in the long run. Try to make one small change each week or two on your way to an improved quality of life. It is extremely difficult to stick to lifestyle modifications if you try many at the same time. It can be much easier if you look toward one improvement; maybe you simply add eating breakfast to your morning routine. Once you have that down for a couple of weeks, incorporate an evening jog three nights a week around the block. Slowly add more to your lifestyle changes as you feel successful in the small things.

Getting and staying fit is the accumulation of daily healthy choices. You should be able to enjoy a decadent piece of birthday cake on an occasion that seems special but try to avoid making food indulgences a regular occurrence. Soon enough, a bowl of tasty guacamole with lots of healthy fats will feel satisfying and like a treat just as much as a piece of candy would. It takes conscious effort but only small changes to see a big difference.

For some people, their eating habits are out of control and small focus for them could be related to nutrition. For others, they tend to struggle getting a regular workout in. If you fall in this category, then I recommend you get a workout partner, join a running club, or sign up for a 5K walk to get you motivated with a time centered goal. It can be extremely overwhelming to look at where you are now and picture where you want to be without any idea how you can get there. Instead of looking at the distance you have to go, take each day and make decisions that can improve your health. You are worth it. Whether you are a mother, father, sister, or friend, your health matters. Reward yourself with something you have been dying to have an excuse to do like getting a massage or spending the day at the beach. You can set a great example to others by making positive changes toward a healthier you.

Be kind to yourself. We are all in a constant state of change. And when we talk about our physical health, it is easy to look at the failures. I encourage you to celebrate in the small things. If you hoped for a thirty-minute run but can go for a ten-minute walk, be happy you did something! Throw out the all-or-nothing thinking and get moving.

If you are struggling to find focus, use this book as a guide but also have the courage to reach out and ask for help. Maybe hiring a trainer for a short amount of time will help get you going or maybe you can sign up for an online weight loss support group. Consider being open with your partner/spouse/friends about how important healthy lifestyle changes are for you. Gaining a team of support around you will strengthen you and increase the likelihood that you will reach your set goals.

It is my sincere hope that this book can serve as a reference with lots of tools to put in your healthy lifestyle toolbox. Some of the weight training and stretching ideas might be a great resource for a last minute workout you can accomplish on your own time. Pick and choose a few of them to perform when you need a short workout. Take advantage of the online and app resources now so readily available. Come back to it every now and then for inspiration and a new idea. Let it be motivation for a new approach to obtaining a healthier life. You will always feel encouraged and healthier by making positive changes toward being the best version of you!

To say the least, I'd love to hear from you! You can write to me at ssimmons@corban.edu. Write soon!

Made in the USA
San Bernardino, CA
07 January 2015